Candida Albicans

Other titles in this series:
High Blood Pressure
Irritable Bowel Syndrome
The Menopause

By the same author:
The Complete Book of Men's Health
High Blood Pressure
Irritable Bowel Syndrome
The Menopause

Dr Sarah Brewer MA, MB, BChir

CANDIDA ALBICANS

Thorsons
An Imprint of HarperCollins*Publishers*

Thorsons
An Imprint of HarperCollins*Publishers*
77–85 Fulham Palace Road,
Hammersmith, London W6 8JB
1160 Battery Street,
San Francisco, California 94111–1213
Published by Thorsons 1997

10 9 8 7 6 5 4 3 2 1

A catalogue record for this book
is available from the British Library

ISBN 0 7225 3391 8

Printed in Great Britain by
Caledonian International Book Manufacturing, Glasgow

To Richard and Saxon

CONTENTS

PREFACE: THE ESSENTIAL GUIDE SERIES

This series offers up-to-date, in-depth information on common health problems. These books contain detailed, medically accurate information in a user-friendly, easy to read style.

Each book covers:

- What the condition is
- How common it is
- Who is affected by it
- Normal body functions and how each condition affects them
- Symptoms
- Causes
- Risk factors
- How the condition is diagnosed – blood tests, investigations, etc.
- Other similar conditions that need to be ruled out
- The drugs used to treat it – including side-effects and who shouldn't take them
- Surgical treatments that can help
- Complementary treatments
- Self-help tips
- Dietary changes that may prove helpful
- Latest research findings
- Addresses of support groups and sources of further information

This invaluable series will answer all your questions and help you to make the best decisions regarding your own health care.

Chapter One

AN INTRODUCTION TO CANDIDA

Not all yeast cells are as accommodating as those that produce the finest vintage champagne. Unlike its cousins, yeasts used in brewing and baking, the yeast known generally as Candida can cause a number of human diseases ranging from nappy rash to lethal meningitis in people with lowered immunity.

At the beginning of the 20th century, infection with Candida was rare. It now seems to be a significant problem for a great number of people. Many researchers believe this is due to wide-spread use of broad-spectrum antibiotics, which disrupt the normal balance of healthy micro-organisms in the body as well as killing disease-causing pathogens. It is also partly because modern medical treatments allow people with serious illnesses and lowered resistance to live longer so they become susceptible to yeast 'super-infections'.

Many apparently healthy people are plagued with recurrent Candida infections despite being otherwise well. Not only is the Candida yeast changing – and perhaps becoming more virulent – but modern lifestyles are also partly to blame. Hormonal methods of contraception, raised stress levels, low-temperature washing machine cycles and a diet of highly processed food are all playing a role. It is also thought that Candida can produce an allergic-type reaction (Candida hypersensitivity syndrome) linked to a number of common conditions such as Irritable Bowel Syndrome and constant fatigue.

WHAT IT IS

Candida is the name for a group of yeast-like fungi that live quite happily in or on the body of just about everyone. They exist in balance with other micro-organisms (commensals) – on the skin, in the intestines and sometimes in the mouth or genital tract – usually without causing any obvious harm.

Altogether, around 80 different species of Candida exist, but only a quarter of these can cause disease in humans. Of these, the most important is *Candida albicans* – or white fungus. It is named after the white plaques that form on mucous membranes in a well-established infection. The common name for Candida infection is thrush.

Candida belong to a large group (division) of fungi that are described as imperfect (*fungi imperfecti*) because they have mostly lost the art of sexual reproduction. Most increase in numbers by growing and putting out little buds that break off and form new daughter cells.

When Candida are viewed under the microscope, they take on several different forms, some of which look like classic yeasts, while others resemble fungi:

- large, round, thick-walled inactive resting spores (chlamydioconidia)
- active yeast cells that may be round, slipper- or pear-shaped
- asexually reproducing yeast cells with budding daughter cells (blastoconidia) projecting from their surface to resemble knobbly Jerusalem artichokes
- a collection of elongated buds and threads that have remained attached to one another rather than breaking off (pseudohyphae)
- long thread-like structures (germ tubes or hyphae)
- a network of interwoven threads (mycelium).

The simple-cell forms of Candida remain superficial and are seen when Candida yeasts colonize the skin, mouth, gut or lower reproductive tract without causing symptoms. The thread forms (hyphae and psudohyphae), however, can burrow down between human cells to literally invade the tissues and cause symptoms of Candida overgrowth.

If Candida proliferates in large numbers or starts to invade the tissues, it produces varying symptoms depending on the part of the body affected and how mild or severe the infection is. These symptoms include:

- itching
- discharge
- soreness
- redness
- painful swelling
- swollen glands
- skin rash
- brittle nails
- difficulty swallowing
- painful intercourse
- cystitis
- weight loss
- lack of energy.

Recurrent Candida infection makes life a misery for countless numbers of people.

Candida infection is also known as:
- Candidiasis
- Candidosis
- Moniliasis
- Thrush

WHERE IT COMES FROM

Candida yeast cells are found just about everywhere on Earth. Because they can enter a resting state similar to suspended animation (spores) they exist even in inhospitable places – including surviving a relatively low-temperature (40°C) cycle in your washing machine. Candida have been recovered from soil, food and also from the air. Most of us carry around our own unique strains of Candida, which cause no problems until our natural immunity is lowered, as during illness (such as a cold) or through taking antibiotics.

HOW COMMON IS IT?

Candida albicans is so common that it lives in or on the body of just about every member of the population. Altogether, it accounts for up to 75 per cent of yeasts recovered from sites of infection. It can also be isolated from normal, healthy individuals with no signs of disease, and is found in:

- the mouths of up to 50 per cent of healthy people
- the oesophagus of 11 per cent of healthy people
- rectal swabs of 30 per cent of healthy people
- vaginal swabs of up to 55 per cent of apparently well women
- the faeces of 80 per cent of healthy people
- the skin creases of up to 80 per cent of healthy people
- the hands of 12 per cent of doctors and nurses
- the mouths of 76 per cent of hospital patients.

Three out of four women experience vaginal thrush at least once in their life; some are plagued with never-ending recurrences.

WHAT TRIGGERS CANDIDA OVERGROWTH?

Candida yeast cells usually live in a happy balance with healthy bacteria and cause no harm. It is only when conditions change, encouraging the overgrowth of yeast cells, that they can invade your tissues and cause symptoms. Its favourite conditions for optimum survival are a warm, moist place with an acid pH (2.5 –7.5) and a temperature of 20 to 38°C – the usual conditions found in the vagina and some parts of the gut. Even when conditions are not ideal, the yeast can still proliferate. In general, a symptomatic Candida infection is most likely to develop if:

- a particularly virulent strain of Candida is present
- local conditions such as temperature, humidity or acid levels

change enough to encourage Candida growth (as after vigorous exercise, after using a vaginal douche, when taking antacids)

■ circulating hormones (especially oestrogens) activate yeast cells (for example, at certain times in the female menstrual cycle and during pregnancy)

■ there is an imbalance of other micro-organisms which usually keep yeast cells in check (for example in the gut or vagina after taking antibiotics)

■ local carbohydrate levels (glycogen or glucose) are increased, providing ideal growing conditions for fungal cells (as in people with diabetes, or in vaginal secretions at certain times of the menstrual cycle)

■ physical or mental stress (for example work stress, surgery, accidents) has lowered a person's natural immunity

■ immune cells are temporarily less efficient at fighting fungal infections (for example because of another illness such as a viral cold, or because of a deficiency of certain vitamins or minerals)

■ natural immunity has been lowered by taking certain drugs (for example steroids, chemotherapy, immune suppressants)

■ immune cells are less efficient at fighting fungal infections because of a serious illness such as cancer or AIDS.

Candida albicans can infect different parts of the body, including:
■ joints (Candidal arthritis) *(see Chapter 3)*
■ skin *(see Chapter 4)*
■ ears *(see Chapter 4)*
■ nappy area *(see Chapter 4)*
■ nails *(see Chapter 4)*
■ bladder (cystitis) *(see Chapter 5)*
■ vulva *(see Chapter 5)*
■ vagina *(see Chapter 5)*
■ mouth *(see Chapter 6)*
■ oesophagus (gullet) *(see Chapter 6)*
■ gut (enteritis) *(see Chapter 6)*
■ lungs (fungus ball pneumonitis) *(see Chapter 7)*
■ lining of the heart (endocarditis) *(see Chapter 7)*
■ lining of the brain (meningitis) *(see Chapter 7)*

- brain (Candidal abscess) *(see Chapter 7)*
- kidneys (pyelonephritis) *(see Chapter 7)*
- blood (septicaemia) *(see Chapter 7)*

The more serious infections only affect patients whose immune system is seriously impaired, for example patients undergoing organ transplants, or those with terminal cancer or AIDS.

Chapter Two

THE NORMAL IMMUNE SYSTEM

To understand how the symptoms of Candida infection develop, it's worth looking at the function of the normal immune system and how it usually fights off infections such as yeasts.

The immune system is made up of millions of armed cells that patrol the body and protect it against disease. These cells can recognize and help to repel:

- foreign invaders such as bacteria, viruses or yeasts
- foreign proteins such as poisons
- infected or cancerous cells
- transplanted foreign tissues.

In order to perform these functions, immune cells have to identify normal components of the body and leave them alone, while at the same time recognizing cells that shouldn't be there. To add to the complexity of their task, they also have to pick out and destroy body cells that have changed in some way – either through infection or another disease process such as cancer.

Each body cell bears surface identity tags that brand it as part of the self. Immune cells learn to recognize these early, during fetal development, and generally leave them alone.

Foreign cells such as bacteria, viruses or Candida cells bear very different cell markers – usually in the form of sugar-protein complexes (glycoproteins) sticking out from their cell walls or membranes. Usually, immune cells instantly recognize these markers (antigens) as foreign and activate the full brunt of their arsenal to engulf or destroy the invaders.

As well as displaying self-markers, body cells continually process and break down internal proteins, fragments of which are transported to the cell membrane and displayed on their surface. This allows each body cell to communicate its internal conditions to circulating immune cells. As soon as an infected or cancerous cell is encountered that bears both a self-hallmark plus foreign markers (for example cells belonging to a virus, or tumour protein), the cell is recognized as undesirable and destroyed.

CELLS INVOLVED IN THE IMMUNE RESPONSE

All the cells involved in your immune responses are derived from common stem cells which develop in the bone marrow or the thymus gland. In general, cells known as B cells are derived from bone marrow, while those referred to as T cells are programmed in the thymus. The thymus is a gland found in the upper part of the chest, behind the sternum. It is relatively large in infancy but starts to shrink at puberty and has virtually disappeared by adulthood, although remnants are often present until middle age.

Immune cells communicate with each other by secreting chemical alarm signals called cytokines. Cytokines are soluble factors that quickly attract other patrolling immune cells into an area and super-stimulate them for a swift immune response. The main cells involved in the immune response are macrophages, neutrophils and lymphocytes.

Macrophages

Macrophage literally means 'big eater'. These are long-lived scavenger cells that patrol all parts of the body. They start their early training in the bloodstream where they have a round, compact shape and are usually referred to as monocytes. When a monocyte encounters signs of trouble, it quickly sticks to the blood vessel wall, contorts itself into a long thin shape and squeezes between the cells in the blood vessel wall to take up residence in the body tissues. It then moves around the body by putting out cell elongations known as pseudopodia, or 'false feet'. It hunts down and envelops unwanted tissue debris, dead or dying cells and foreign invaders. Once it has identified a bacterium, virus, yeast or infected body cell, it secretes a chemical 'siren' in the form of cytokines which quickly attract other immune cells into the area. At the same time, the macrophage absorbs foreign proteins (antigens) from the unwanted cell on to its surface and presents these to the circulating lymphocytes to super-stimulate them. Macrophages are particularly concentrated in the liver, spleen and in the lymph nodes dotted throughout the lymphatic system. They even take up residence in tissues such as the brain, where they are known as microglial cells, and inside calcified bone, where they are known as osteoclasts and help to dissolve and remodel old bone tissue.

Neutrophils

Neutrophils make up around 60 per cent of circulating white blood cells and are more commonly known as pus cells. These only live for 6–20 hours but play a vital role against infection and disease – their absence usually proves fatal. They are attracted into areas of infection and inflammation by cytokines. Once there, they literally eat invading micro-organisms such as bacteria by enveloping them and pulling them inside their cell membrane (phagocytosis). A lethal bag of chemicals (containing toxic hydrogen peroxide among others) is then quickly emptied onto the invader to kill it. Neutrophils also have special receptors on their cell surface that can interact with antibodies or special protein bombs (complement – *see below*) to speed up the process of destruction. With larger invaders such as Candida yeast cells, neutrophils can stick to them and release chemicals that damage the cells sufficiently to put them out of action. Neutrophils carry around their own energy stores in the form of a starchy glycogen. This means they can penetrate inhospitable areas (for example the middle of an abscess) and still survive long enough to do damage despite lack of other nutrients or oxygen.

Lymphocytes

Lymphocytes make up around 40 per cent of circulating white blood cells. There are three different types which are recognized by their different surface markers and different patterns of activity:

1. Natural Killer (NK) cells (10 per cent of total lymphocytes)
2. B lymphocytes (20 per cent of total; derived from the bone marrow)
3. T lymphocytes (70 per cent of total; derived from the thymus).

Natural Killer Cells

These are mainly concerned with killing abnormal body cells which are infected with a virus or which have turned cancerous. They are super-stimulated by tissue macrophages and provide an important first line of defence while the more specific T and B lymphocytes power themselves into action. Rather like a kamikaze pilot, the NK cell usually dies during its attack.

B Lymphocytes

These make antibodies. You inherit many different families or lines of B cells, each of which makes one – and only one – specific antibody aimed against a particular foreign protein (antigen). A number of these identical antibodies stick out from the surface of the B lymphocyte rather like the weapons on a Dalek. Until it is activated, a B lymphocyte patrols the body in low numbers, in an armed but inactive form known as a B memory cell. When a foreign antigen enters the body, it encounters a dazzling array of different B lymphocytes, only one or two of which bear the right antibodies to recognize and react to its foreign proteins. As soon as the B lymphocyte encounters the foreign protein against which its antibody is directed, it powers up and starts to produce large numbers of its single, specific antibody. These active, bristling lymphocytes are known as B plasma cells. Their activity is regulated by various T lymphocytes, which act like administrators to control, encourage or inhibit their various activities. During activation, the B plasma cell divides repeatedly to build up a sub-population of cells producing a particular type of antibody. Once the invasion is over, there will be many more B lymphocyte memory cells for this particular type patrolling your body. If the same invader is encountered again, your immune response will be that much quicker and angrier, making it less easy for the organism to gain a foothold.

T lymphocytes

These exist in several different forms, some of which interact with B lymphocytes to regulate antibody production:

- T helper cells – help to power up B memory cells and stimulate them into making antibody
- T suppresser cells – bring antibody production to a halt (as when an infection has been beaten)
- T cytotoxic (killer) cells – more sophisticated versions of the natural killer cells which tend to survive their attacks and go on to assassinate other targets.
- T delayed hypersensitivity cells – involved in some hypersensitivity (allergic) reactions.

Antibodies

Antibodies, or immunoglobulins, are soluble glycoproteins (made from sugar and protein molecules) present throughout body fluids. They are produced by activated B lymphocytes, each of which produces only one type of antibody.

An antibody is made up of four protein chains: two identical heavy (long) chains and two identical light (short) chains, that link together to form a Y-shaped molecule.

When an antibody encounters a foreign antigen (for example a surface marker on a yeast cell) that it is directed against, the open end of the Y-shaped antibody clamps on to the antigen, making the cellular equivalent of a citizen's arrest. The antibody's tail chain sticks out behind and waits for help to arrive in the form of a macrophage, neutrophil, natural killer cell, cytotoxic T lymphocyte or a protein bomb (complement – *see page 12*). This extra help homes in on the antibody-antigen complex and quickly destroys it.

Antibodies are divided into five different classes depending on the type of heavy chain they contain:

1. IgA – a double antibody made of two identical antibodies joined tail to tail; mainly secreted into fluids on body linings and surfaces, for example into sweat, tears, saliva, intestinal juices, vaginal secretions; one of its main functions is to interfere with the binding of organisms such as Candida to body cells, so preventing them from invading the body
2. IgD – seems to play a role in controlling the activation and powering down of B lymphocytes
3. IgE – involved in triggering inflammation to produce a rapid immune response – unfortunately, this often misfires and produces an allergic response, for example the release of histamine when pollen grains land in the nose or eyes
4. IgG – the main type of circulating, protective antibody which neutralizes toxins and helps to wipe out invaders
5. IgM – a complex made of five antibodies joined together to form a star shape; they are largely confined to the bloodstream and are highly affective at trapping and immobilizing invaders.

Complement

The complement system is a series of around 20 circulating proteins that stick to antigen-antibody complexes in a specific sequence. As the different proteins link up, like part of a jigsaw, they eventually form a powerful enzyme. This acts rather like a protein bomb to blow up and destroy an antibody–antigen complex or an invading organism – complement can literally blow holes in the side of a bacterium or yeast cell to kill it.

The Lymph System

The body contains an extensive network of lymph vessels which drain every tissue in the body. Fluid that passes out of the blood bathes the cells and forms what is known as the internal sea. This fluid provides your cells with nutrients and flushes away wastes resulting from cell metabolism. The fluid also contains salts and dissolved immune chemicals such as antibodies, cytokines and complement, and is patrolled by billions of immune cells. Fluids from the internal sea are drained away through lymph vessels which filter it through a series of lymph nodes (sometimes known as glands) before returning it to your veins. Each lymph node varies from 1–20 mm in diameter and contains a series of channels packed full of macrophages plus lymphocytes armed with antibodies. Any debris or infection (for example yeast cells) present in the fluid drained from your tissues is filtered out by the sieve-like action of the lymph nodes and promptly attacked and destroyed by the immune cells present.

WHEN CANDIDA STRIKES

In order to cause symptoms, Candida must first get a hold in part of the body and evade the normal immune defences.

Sticking

The first step in an attack of Candida occurs when yeast cells stick to the mucous membrane cells, for example in the mouth, gut, vulva or vagina. They do this by using special receptors on their outer cell wall (the so-called fuzzy coat) which act rather like suckers or NASA landing equipment. Some species of Candida (for example *Candida albicans*, *C. tropicalis*) stick to epithelial (lining) cells more easily than others and are therefore more likely to cause disease. The ability to stick also depends on local conditions, such as temperature and acidity levels.

Growing

Once the yeast cells have obtained an anchorage on the host cell they start to develop germ tubes (hyphae) which coat the surface of the host cells. As the Candida yeast cells bud, increase in numbers and put out hyphae, they may form a raised white plaque resembling a curd of cottage cheese.

Dissolving

The next stage in causing an attack comes when the hyphae start to secrete enzymes that can break down protein (such as collagen) and fats. The enzymes loosen and dissolve connections between the host cell membranes and let the hyphae burrow their way down between layers of cells to penetrate quite deeply. The hyphae can actually penetrate inside your cells, from which they steal nutrients and energy. The main body of the yeast may remain attached to the epithelial surface (the lining of the gut, vagina etc.) or it may slip inside one of your cells. This is thought to be one way in which some yeast infections manage to evade your immune defences, hide from anti-fungal drugs and pop up again and again to cause infection. The species of Candida that produce the most enzymes (such as *C. albicans*) are the ones most likely to produce symptoms and signs of infection. This enzyme activity is also responsible for some of the soreness and inflammation that accompanies an attack of thrush.

Switching

Smooth colonies of Candida yeast cells growing in cell cultures can switch to producing colonies with an uneven, rough surface when exposed to low doses of ultraviolet light. The switched (rough) colonies produce different patterns of germ tube threads (hyphae), and seem to:

- stick to body lining cells more easily
- proliferate more readily
- secrete more enzymes that break down proteins, fats and cell walls
- be more invasive
- escape from detection by immune cells more easily
- be less susceptible to anti-fungal treatments.

Translocation

The gut is the main site from which Candida yeasts enter the body. This is known as translocation (moving across). Live yeast cells can enter the circulation from anywhere in the bowel, but the most likely source seems to be a part of the small intestine called the jejunum. When only a small number of yeast cells are involved, these are usually quickly mopped up by macrophage scavenger cells – it is only when large numbers of Candida cells are involved, or where the immune system is seriously weakened, that Candida can invade deeper body tissues. Candida can also enter the circulation from the lungs, though this is thought to account for less than 3 per cent of systemic Candida infections.

Invasion

Occasionally, if the immune system is very weak Candida can set up colonies deep in body tissues to form micro-abscesses. This causes serious, even potentially lethal problems (for example Candidal brain abscess, meningitis, fungus ball pneumonia, etc.) and is known as systemic Candidiasis.

HOW THE IMMUNE SYSTEM FIGHTS CANDIDA INFECTIONS

Most yeast infections are kept at bay by a fine balance between the strength of your immune system and the virulence (ability to cause disease) of the strains of Candida living in and on your body. In the majority of cases, Candida benignly colonizes your body without causing harm. It is only when there is a breakdown in your normal defences that Candida strikes, acting as a disease-causing organism (opportunistic pathogen).

Your Skin

Your outer layer of skin forms a hardened (cornified) physical barrier. It is made up of dead skin cells that have been transformed into armoured plates of the tough protein, keratin. These plates are regularly sloughed and replaced, so that any yeast cells sticking to them are lost from the outer surface of the body. Fats (lipids) present in skin sweat and oils also seem to inhibit the growth of Candida cells. The usual cause of a Candida infection taking hold on the skin is a breach in skin integrity, for example a wound, burn, exposure to excessive moisture (maceration) or the presence of another disease such as eczema. This is one reason why Candida infections are likely to infect skin folds (for example in the nappy region) – a build-up of warmth, moisture and chemicals in sweat makes the skin boggy so that Candida can take hold. For a similar reason, Candida infection of the hand may occur in people whose hands are often wet (for example dishwashers) and in children who regularly suck their thumb.

Your Mucous Membranes

The mucous membranes lining your mouth, gut, respiratory and genito-urinary tracts are less well defended than your outer skin and are therefore more susceptible to Candida infection. These body surfaces are warm, moist places – exactly the sort of sites where Candida loves to stick and grow. Subtle changes in the local environment can tip the balance so that symptoms of infection occur.

In the mouth, some protection is provided by the continual flushing with saliva that contains enzymes, chemicals and antibodies, mainly of the double antibody type IgA which inhibit Candida growth. Factors which increase the risk of mouth yeast infections include having mouth ulcers, smoking cigarettes, wearing dentures, using inhaled steroid preparations (as to treat asthma) and having raised blood sugar levels in diabetes. Experiments also show that sheer numbers of Candida cells can cause infection – a volunteer who drank a solution containing 1,000,000,000,000 Candida cells developed Candidosis of the gut; live yeast cells were later isolated from his bloodstream and urine.

Secretions in the oesophagus (gullet) and intestines also contain enzymes, antibodies (mainly antibody type IgA) and infection-fighting cells (macrophages, neutrophils, lymphocytes). Taking oral corticosteroid tablets, antibiotics or treatments to suppress stomach acid production (for example when peptic ulcers are present) can all increase the chance of Candida taking hold and causing problems in some people. Similarly, those using inhaled steroids are also more likely to develop oesophageal Candidiasis.

Tissue Fluids

After your skin or mucous membrane barriers have been breached by Candidal cells, your next line of defence consists of the immune factors present in your tissue fluids (the internal sea). These include complement and antibodies. These factors coat invading yeast cells and hasten their destruction by immune cells. The presence of too much antibody may coat the yeast cells so well that they are hidden from attacking immune cells, however, and paradoxically this may help to keep the infection going. Some people also develop an allergic response if they have made antibody of the IgE type, which can make symptoms of Candidiasis worse.

Immune Cells

Your most important final line of defence against Candidiasis is made up of the pus cells (neutrophils) and scavenger cells (macrophages in the tissues and monocytes in the blood) that roam your body and attack invaders. Lack of neutrophils – for example in some people with leukaemia – or a default in neutrophil function (present in some people with inherited enzyme defects) makes the risk of widespread Candidiasis much higher. Dying neutrophils that have been overwhelmed by an infection also release chemicals which either damage yeast cells or interfere with their function by mopping up the mineral zinc ions which the yeast cell needs for its metabolism.

Inflammation

Most of the symptoms associated with an attack of thrush are due to the inflammatory reactions set up as part of your body's natural immune defences. Macrophages patrolling your tissues come across fungal hyphae and instantly recognize something is wrong. They start trying to eat the invaders and send out chemical alarm signals (cytokines) which quickly attract other macrophages, neutrophils and lymphocytes into the area. Circulating antibodies may also bind to the hyphae and attract immune cells and complement proteins, making the immune response more effective.

As a result of tissue damage by thrush cells, and the chemicals released by the body to fight off the infection, local blood vessels (capillaries) dilate and leak clear blood fluids (plasma) into the area. This brings in extra complement protein and extra antibodies, and makes it easier for immune cells to slip through the blood vessel walls. This dilation of blood vessels results in the increased warmth, redness and swelling that accompanies inflammation. The chemicals also irritate nerve-endings to cause pain. This is why a thrush infection of the mouth, vagina or vulva, for example, can be so uncomfortable.

Altering Your Defences

There is evidence that chemicals made by yeasts can alter the normal immune response which keeps infection at bay. Substances released by the hyphae and pseudohyphae of *Candida albicans*, and present in their cell walls, have been found to increase susceptibility to certain bacterial infections (for example Staphylococci and Streptococci). These substances damp down the activity of neutrophils (pus cells) so that they:

- are less likely to be attracted into the area
- move more sluggishly
- are less able to engulf and absorb fungal cells
- are less able to bombard absorbed fungal products with a bag of toxic chemicals.

Other fungal products seem to impair activity of T lymphocytes so that they don't react to the presence of Candida cells, in which case a long-term (chronic) infection is more likely to occur.

Allergic Reactions

Some people are particularly sensitive to Candida infections as they have circulating antibodies of the IgE type which respond to Candida proteins. IgE can trigger release of histamine and other allergy chemicals from cells. They may also have T lymphocytes sensitized against yeast cells. These trigger an over-reaction and keep inflammatory reactions powered up to cause excessive redness, pain and swelling. They may also be associated with chronic inflammatory reactions which can lead to feelings of tiredness all the time and lack of energy (*see* Candida Hypersensitivity Syndrome, *pages 22 and 91*).

Predisposing Factors for a Single Attack of Candida

- antibiotics
- stress
- hormone levels – periods, pregnancy

Predisposing Factors for Recurrent Candida

- low ferritin levels *(see page 57)*
- high blood sugar levels in diabetes
- nutritional deficiencies: lack of vitamins and minerals

Factors that May Increase Your Risk of Candidiasis

- exposure to large numbers of Candida cells
- being overtired, run-down, physically unfit or under another form of stress
- having another infection that ties up your immune system and weakens it (for example influenza)
- taking treatments that suppress stomach acid production (for example antacids)
- using inhaled corticosteroids (for example for asthma), which damp down immune reactions in the mouth and respiratory tract
- taking oral corticosteroid therapy, which damps down immune reactions throughout the body
- having a serious illness that weakens the immune system (for example cancer)
- having treatment that damps down the immune system (for example chemotherapy, radiotherapy)
- poor nutrition and weight loss
- tissue damage (for example cuts, burns, ulcers, tooth extraction)
- smoking cigarettes
- wearing dentures

Chapter Three

SYMPTOMS AND SIGNS OF CANDIDA INFECTION

So many symptoms seem to be triggered by Candida – either through an overgrowth of the yeasts or as a result of hypersensitivity to them – that it is easy for sufferers to be dismissed by their doctor, family and colleagues as suffering from hypochondria or a neurotic problem. This is especially true if symptoms come and go or change, as they often do. While some people will only suffer mild nuisance symptoms which do not interfere unduly with their life, others are debilitated by constant tiredness and non-specific feelings of being unwell. This interferes with concentration, quality and quantity of work output and can make you so irritable and depressed that it jeopardizes relationships at home and at work.

The symptoms you might experience depend on where the Candida infection has struck. You may only develop a few of the symptoms listed here, or may suffer from the lot:

Skin	itchiness/soreness/redness/scaly rash/flakiness/acne-like spots
Skin folds	itchiness/soreness/redness/maceration (moist breakdown of skin)/weeping sores/build-up of white clots
Nappy area	generalized redness involving skin creases/soreness/weeping areas/red spots (satellite lesions) outside main affected area/possible build-up of white clots

Nails	unsightly ridges/brittleness, flaking, splitting/ discoloration of nail plate/soreness around edge of nails (paronychia)
Mouth	coated tongue/bad breath (halitosis)/itching (for example on the roof of the mouth, beneath dentures)/redness/soreness/dryness (xerostomia)/pain on eating or drinking/ white plaques on inside of mouth/ulceration cracks at corners of mouth
Oesophagus	difficulty or pain on swallowing/pain behind the breastbone (retrosternal)/nausea, vomiting/bringing up blood (haematemesis)/ sometimes fever
Intestinal tract	sensitivity to certain foods/pain on swallowing/heartburn, indigestion, flatulence, bloating/diarrhoea/constipation
Anal area	intense itching/soreness/moist discharge/ weeping sores/difficulty or pain on opening the bowels/worsening of symptoms due to piles
Female reproductive tract (vaginitis/vulvitis)	itching/redness/soreness/dryness/a white, cottage-cheese-like discharge/pain on intercourse/cystitis-like pain on passing urine (dysuria)/frequency of urination/enlarged lymph nodes (glands) in the groin
Male reproductive tract (balanitis)	mild itching on end of penis/soreness of end of penis/red spots/white plaques/build-up of white material under the foreskin/pain on passing urine (dysuria)/enlarged lymph nodes (glands) in the groin

CAUSES

When Candida cells change from their simple cell form to the activated form, threads of fungal material (germ tubes, or hyphae) burrow down between mucous membrane cells lining your mouth, gut, vagina, end of the penis or around the anus. This causes small areas of ulceration and fissuring which exposes tiny, sensitive nerve-endings.

Some of the threads also puncture straight through your cells, releasing powerful intra-cellular enzymes into surrounding tissues. This starts up the inflammatory response which attracts immune cells into the area. Yet more chemicals are released into the inflamed tissues as blood vessels dilate, so the area swells and becomes sore. These chemicals irritate the already raw nerve-endings and you may experience pain and throbbing sensations depending on how bad the infection is and where it has struck.

This inflammation due to your normal immune response to infection causes symptoms of redness, swelling, tenderness and throbbing pain. Local lymph nodes (glands) may also be swollen.

As well as specific symptoms linked to the site of infection, you may also develop non-specific symptoms linked with Candida Hypersensitivity Syndrome:

- fatigue
- tiredness all the time
- lethargy and disinterest
- malaise
- dizziness
- irritability
- anxiety
- depression
- insomnia
- difficulty concentrating
- headache
- joint and muscle pain
- poor appetite
- cravings for sugar and carbohydrate

- recurrent cystitis where no evidence of infection is found
- Irritable Bowel Syndrome
- alcohol intolerance
- problems after taking antibiotics.

Chapter Four

FUNGAL INFECTIONS OF THE SKIN

Fungal skin infections vary from widespread dry rashes to single scaly patches or moist, boggy areas. Single lesions are often known as ringworm, as they can form rings with a raised edge that spread outwards as the centre clears and returns to normal. There is no worm involved, however, only a fungus of which three types are the main culprits:

1. Candida yeasts
2. Pityrosporum yeasts
3. Dermatophytes.

Symptoms vary and can include:

- itchiness
- diffuse redness in skin folds, usually with a distinct edge
- beefy, red, slightly raised areas of swelling in skin folds
- white thrush-like plaques
- discrete ring-like red lesions (ringworm)
- small satellite lesions spreading away from the main area of infection
- scaling
- enlarging red lesions with a raised, irregular edge
- widespread inflammation of hair follicles (folliculitis)
- burning soreness
- painful cracking
- oozing sores
- loss of skin (desquamation)
- pink-brown patches

- depigmented white areas
- patches of hair loss.

Other skin conditions can be mistaken for fungal infections, and vice versa. These include eczema, psoriasis, and even some forms of skin cancer (for example squamous cell carcinoma). If you think you have a fungal skin infection which has not responded to treatment within a couple of weeks, or which seems to be getting worse rather than better, it is important to seek medical advice.

CANDIDA SKIN INFECTIONS

Candida skin infections only usually occur if the skin is damaged by a build-up of moistness (for example in skin folds, within your shoes), by burns or friction or where there is an existing skin problem such as eczema. It is more common in people with diabetes, those taking antibiotics and where the immune system is weakened by another disease. When Candida infection does strike, it frequently affects skin folds such as those in:

- the groin
- the armpits
- under the breasts
- between the toes or fingers (Athlete's foot)
- in the groin (tinea cruris)
- around the scrotum or penis (balanitis)
- around the vaginal entrance (vulvo-vaginitis)
- under rolls of fat, for example on the abdomen
- between the buttocks in adults
- the nappy area in babies.

These areas are warm, moist places where yeast cells thrive quite happily. In 8 out of 10 cases, *Candida albicans* is responsible as this type of yeast seems to stick to the outer, toughened skin scales (keratinocytes) more easily than other Candida species. The infection usually stays confined to the upper skin layers, but where the immune system is weakened, or damage to the skin has penetrated into deep layers, it may penetrate further into tissues to cause more severe symptoms.

Careful hygiene is needed – especially in warm summer months – to prevent a build-up of acid, sweaty skin secretions which can damage the skin (maceration) and allow Candida or other skin fungi to take hold. Classic lesions have the appearance of white clots on a bright red background.

Candida can also cause inflammation of hair follicles (folliculitis) with small raised red pimples/pustules surrounding tiny hairs on the skin. This usually occurs under occlusive dressings that have become wet with sweat (for example plaster casts, bandages) and can also be triggered by shaving near infected areas. This condition is known as *Candida miliaria* or 'heat rash', and is also linked with profuse sweating. The yeast infection may be mistaken for similar symptoms caused by bacteria or inflammation (for example pustular eczema) and may get worse if the wrong treatment (for example antibiotics) is given.

PITYROSPORUM YEAST INFECTIONS

Pityrosporum yeasts are similar to Candida yeasts, but are normally found only on the scalp. Like Candida, they usually live on the skin quite happily as commensal organisms without causing problems. If they proliferate excessively, however, they can trigger skin flaking, dandruff and – in babies – cradle cap (*see page 32*). These conditions are known medically as seborrhoeic capitis, which literally means greasy inflammation of the head. If the infection is left untreated it may spread onto the face, skin flexures or chest to produce a more inflamed skin reaction known as seborrhoeic dermatitis.

On the face, the red, scaly rash commonly affects the eyebrows and forehead, with greasy scaling of the skin folds running between the nose and lips. In people with depressed immunity this may lead to a severe, widespread inflammation of the hair follicles (folliculitis) producing small, itchy, raised lumps (papules).

Under certain circumstances, especially hot, sweaty conditions, Pityrosporum yeasts (especially *Pityrosporum orbiculare*) change to produce fungal-like hyphae similar to those produced by Candida yeasts. This form of the yeast is known as *Malassezia furfur* and causes a characteristic skin rash known as *Pityriasis versicolor*.

The word *pityriasis* comes from the Greek for *bran*, while *versicolor* means of *variable colour*. This fungal infection produces fine, bran-like scales on the skin surface. These cover numerous round or oval patches which are initially pale pink or brown in colour. They gradually become depigmented, to leave white areas that may only show up after exposure to sun, when surrounding uninfected skin becomes tanned. Pityriasis versicolor is often widespread and may be distressing in people with dark skins. The lesions may persist for some time after successful treatment.

DERMATOPHYTES

Dermatophytes are fungal organisms that constantly produce a network of thread-like growths (hyphae). In comparison, yeasts living happily on the skin as commensals usually exist as simple budding cells and only put out germ cell tubes (hyphae) when actively invading your tissues. The dermatophyte hyphae can invade the thickened, outer superficial (keratinized) layers of your hair, skin and nails, but generally only produce mild symptoms. In people suffering from a severely weakened immune system – either as a result of serious illness or some drug treatments – the hyphae can penetrate more deeply into the body.

Three main species of fungus produce dermatophyte infections in humans:

1. Trichophyton rubrum – by far the commonest
2. Trichophyton interdigitalae
3. Epidermophyton floccosum

These dermatophytes affect different parts of the body to produce lesions that are named after the site on which they occur, for example:

- tinea capitis (fungal infection of the scalp)
- tinea pedis (fungal infection of the foot/athlete's foot)
- tinea corporis (fungal infection of the trunk)
- tinea cruris (fungal infection of the groin)
- tinea manuum (fungal infection of the hands)
- onychomycosis (fungal infection of the nails)

The term *tinea* just refers to a fungal infection. Skin fungal infections can also be caught from animals (zoophilic infections). These include fungus spread from cats and dogs (for example *Microsporum canis*), from cattle (for example *Trichophyton verrucusum*) and rodents (such as *Trichophyton mentagrophytes*). These zoophilic infections tend to produce either:

- dry skin infections such as scaling patches of hair loss (alopecia) on the scalp or ring-like scaly lesions (ringworm) on the trunk or limbs
- moist, inflamed, boggy, pustular swellings usually due to cattle ringworm and known as kerions.

Investigation

If you think you have ringworm, it is important to consult your doctor as several other skin problems can cause similar symptoms. Ideally, skin fungal infections need to be confirmed from skin scrapings, as several skin conditions can mimic fungal infection. Skin scrapings, nail clippings or plucked hairs are collected, placed in a fold of black paper and sent to a laboratory for analysis. Examination under a microscope will confirm a dermatophyte or yeast infection. If identification of a particular dermatophyte is important (for example if it may be an infection caught from an animal), the fungus has to be cultured to produce vegetative spores (conidia), as each species has spores of a distinctive shape.

In folliculitis (infection of hair follicles) a Candida or a bacterial infection are told apart by opening and swabbing a fresh pustule, examining it under a microscope for fungi or bacteria and by growing organisms in the laboratory.

Treatment

Localized areas of skin infection can be treated by applying an anti-fungal cream. If the area is very moist (for example under the armpit or breasts), an anti-fungal powder can be used separately, or applied after the cream.

- Clotrimazole cream/powder: applied 2 or 3 times a day and continued for 2 weeks after symptoms have gone
- Miconazole cream/spray/powder: twice a day and continued for 10 days after healing
- Econazole cream: 2 or 3 times a day and continued for 10 days after healing
- Tolnaftate cream/powder/aerosol: twice a day
- Sulconazole cream (prescription only): massaged in twice a day and continued for 2–3 weeks after healing
- Terbinafine cream (prescription only): massaged in once or twice a day for 2–4 weeks.
- Amorolfine cream (prescription only): once daily in the evening for 2–3 weeks, continued for 3–5 days after healing
- Nystatin cream/ointment/gel (prescription only): 2–4 times a day until 1 week after healing

Combined anti-fungal and anti-bacterial treatments may be used where a mixed infection is suspected, for example:

- polynoxylin cream
- nystatin/chlorhexidine cream.

If an underlying inflammatory skin problem such as eczema is suspected, then a combined anti-fungal and anti-inflammatory (corticosteroid) cream may be needed. These are usually only available on prescription (for example clotrimazole and 1 per cent hydrocortisone cream, or the stronger clotrimazole and betamethasone cream) – although preparations containing some of the drug separately (for example 1 per cent clotrimazole or 1 per cent hydrocortisone) are available over the counter.

If a fungal skin infection is mistaken for eczema, and only a plain steroid cream used to treat it (for example 1 per cent hydrocortisone or betamethasone) a condition known as *tinea incognita* (hidden fungal infection) occurs. The steroid cream damps down redness, scaling and itching so that the lesions feel better, but the underlying fungal infection continues to thrive so that skin lesions persist and grow larger – sometimes quite quickly. As soon as treatment is stopped, the infection will return with a vengeance. It is only when an anti-fungal agent is used that the skin infection will get better.

Treating Pityriasis Versicolor

Mild cases of the skin infection pityriasis versicolor, can be treated by using a selenium sulphide shampoo on the skin every day while showering or bathing.

It may take a while for the skin colour change to clear, especially if you are tanned. More advanced cases will usually respond to topical anti-fungal creams or – if widespread – to an anti-fungal drug taken by mouth:

- Ketoconazole cream (prescription only; available at NHS expense for people with seborrhoeic dermatitis or pityriasis versicolor). All areas of the body from the neck down to the elbows and knees should be treated. Used once or twice a day.
- Itraconazole capsules: 2 capsules once a day for 7 days. If treating a fungal skin infection other than pityriasis, it may be prescribed at a dose of 1 capsule a day for 15–30 days.
- Terbinafine tablets: 1 a day for 4 weeks
- Griseofulvin tablets: 1–4 times a day for varying lengths of time depending on response – absorption is improved if taken after a fatty meal.

Prevention

- Take steps to prevent excessive sweating, for example by using an aluminium chloride hexahydrate anti-perspirant (*see page 31*).
- Wash, shower or bathe every day to remove acidic, sweaty secretions from skin folds.

- Dry your skin thoroughly after washing.
- Wear loose-fitting clothes made from natural rather than man-made fibres.
- Spray an anti-fungal powder spray in skin folds prone to excessive sweating.
- Don't share towels, flannels or bath sponges.

Excessive Sweating

Everyone has around 3 million sweat glands, of which there are two different types:

1. Eccrine glands, which open directly onto the skin surface
2. Apocrine glands, which open into hair follicles rather than the skin.

Eccrine glands are found all over the skin, but are concentrated on the palms and the soles of the feet. They mainly secrete water and salts during overheating and exercise. This sweat is designed to cool the body down, although high humidity (for example hot, sticky summer weather, conditions inside the average pair of trainers) will interfere with evaporation of sweat and lead to stickiness, embarrassing wetness and an increased tendency to fungal skin infections.

Apocrine glands only develop at puberty and are found in the armpits and groin. As well as secreting water and salts, they also produce fatty acids which are broken down by bacteria to cause the unpleasant smells characteristic of body odour.

Some people suffer from excessive sweating all year round – a condition known as hyperhydrosis. This is due to overactivity of nerve-endings and can also be brought on by anxiety or stress. The main areas to be affected are the armpits, groin, palms, soles of the feet or forehead.

If you suffer from problem perspiration, a 20 per cent solution of aluminium chloride hexahydrate can now be bought over the counter. Until recently this was only available on prescription. When applied to problem areas it enters the sweat glands to form a gel matrix which reduces, then stops the flow of water. The solution should be applied to clean, dry skin at night – when sweat glands are inactive – and washed off the next morning. As excessive sweating comes under control, you will only need to use it once or twice a week.

CANDIDA EAR INFECTIONS

The external ear canal and behind the ear flap are common sites for Candida skin infections, especially in babies. This can produce symptoms of:

- itching
- flaking skin
- soreness
- weeping behind the ears
- discharge from the ear which often smells unpleasant
- white clots seen inside the ear canal.

Once the diagnosis is made, a Candida ear infection can usually be quickly treated with ear drops containing anti-fungal drugs such as clioquinol (stains skin and clothing) or clotrimazole. Drops should be applied two to three times a day and continued until at least 14 days after symptoms have disappeared.

SCALP YEAST INFECTIONS

Scalp yeast infections affect everyone at some time in life – either as a baby or later, when dandruff can cause great social embarrassment.

Cradle Cap

Mottling and redness of the scalp are common in infants during the first few days and weeks of life. This results from changes in the baby's circulation once he or she adapts to independent life. At the same time, the baby's skin – which was sterile inside the womb – is getting used to being colonized by relatively harmless organisms including skin bacteria and Candida yeasts. This may trigger a mild inflammatory reaction, with redness, dryness and flakiness. Hair follicles may also become more pronounced and pimply.

The skin on the scalp is often affected as bacteria and yeasts take up residence. In most cases only a few flakes develop which quickly fall away. In severe cases, a thick circle of yellow, waxy deposits or crusts builds up, resembling a crocheted hat. This is commonly known as cradle cap and usually appears after the age of 1 month.

Cradle cap is harmless but is a common cause of distress for new mothers. It is a form of seborrhoeic dermatitis whose exact cause is unknown, although it is thought to be a reaction to an overgrowth of the yeast *Pityrosporum ovale*. As well as affecting the scalp, it can also appear on the face, neck, behind the ears and in the nappy area. The skin in these areas may also look red and inflamed.

Sometimes, patches of cradlecap become super-infected by other skin organisms such as Candida or the bacteria Streptococcus or Staphylococcus.

Treatment

Cradle cap is a self-limiting condition and will eventually go away on its own, without treatment, within a few months. This process can be speeded up by a few simple measures:

- Loosen the scales by gently rubbing the scalp with a simple baby shampoo, cetrimide solution, baby oil, olive oil or arachis oil to encourage early sloughing.
- Olive oil or arachis oil can be rubbed into the affected area, left overnight, and then washed off the following day along with the loosened crusts.
- After several days of treatment, most scales should have fallen away. Brushing the hair with a clean soft-bristled brush will help.
- It is important to avoid scratching or picking at affected skin or exposing it to irritants such as detergents. This can lead to inflammation or infection.
- Adding drops of Evening Primrose Oil (EPO) to your baby's feed – or rubbing directly onto affected areas – often results in dramatic improvement. EPO contains an essential fatty

acid – gammalinolenic acid – needed as a building-block for skin cell membranes (*see page 139*). Paediatric capsules with elongated, snippable tops are available, as is a dropper bottle containing pure Evening Primrose Oil.

If the cradle cap is widespread with red inflamed skin that spreads to the armpits, behind the neck and in the nappy area, the baby will need to be checked by a doctor and prescribed the correct treatment for seborrhoeic dermatitis: emollients (skin-softening agents) plus 1 per cent hydrocortisone cream (a mild anti-inflammatory steroid) to reduce any inflammation and redness.

If the skin looks very angry or starts to weep, swabs will need to be sent off for analysis. Anti-Candida creams (for example clotrimazole) or antibiotics may also be needed. If your baby becomes unwell and shows signs of a temperature, goes off his or her food, or seems in any way unwell, obtain medical advice immediately.

Adult Dandruff

Dandruff – dry, flaky skin on the scalp – is a common and annoying problem that affects over 40 per cent of people at some time in their life. It tends to start in adolescence and, unfortunately, once established may be persistent and return once treatment is stopped.

The skin on the scalp is made of normal skin cells that are continually replacing themselves, like skin elsewhere on the body. Dead cells that fall off are usually washed or brushed away without any problem. If the cells are replaced at a faster rate than normal, or if the scalp is excessively dry or greasy, dead cells may clump together to form larger, visible flakes.

The usual cause is a condition known as seborrhoeic dermatitis which produces an itchy, scaly rash on the scalp. Sometimes other areas such as the eyebrows, beard, chest, back and even the groin are affected too, and the skin in these areas may look red and inflamed. Dry or greasy scales may form around the hairline, and in severe cases, a yellowish-red crust appears.

Both mild dandruff and seborrhoeic dermatitis are thought to be triggered by hypersensitivity to the Candida-like yeast,

Pityrosporum. Everyone has small quantities of this yeast on their skin, but in people with scaly scalp problems it may be present in large numbers.

Other conditions that can trigger dandruff include neurodermatitis (stress-related skin scaling), contact dermatitis (for example due to an allergy to ingredients in a shampoo), eczema, psoriasis and sunburn. If your dandruff doesn't clear up within 2 weeks of using an anti-fungal shampoo, don't be embarrassed to consult your doctor as you may have a skin problem needing treatment that is only available on prescription.

Treatment

For mild dandruff, regular shampooing with a gentle product designed for daily use may be enough to clear the condition.

Anti-fungal ingredients reduce flaking and help to control the number of yeast cells present. There are a wide range of shampoos available; different ones work best on different people – experiment until you find one that controls your problem. Shampoos that can clear moderate dandruff contain different active ingredients such as coal tar, zinc pyrithione and selenium sulphide. For more severe problems, a more powerful anti-fungal agent such as ketoconazole will usually work rapidly – until recently this was only available on prescription, but it can now be bought from pharmacies.

If over-the-counter treatments do not clear symptoms within a week or two, or if they are more widespread, consult your doctor as stronger products are available on prescription. Occasionally, dandruff is due to another skin problem such as psoriasis or ringworm, which needs to be properly diagnosed and treated.

Prevention

Wash hair regularly, at least twice a week, to help prevent a build-up of yeast cells and grease.

Use an anti-fungal treatment shampoo once a week, using normal shampoos in between.

Lack of the following nutrients has been linked with adult scaly skin problems:

- vitamin A
- vitamin B$_2$
- vitamin B$_3$
- biotin
- vitamin C
- iodine
- manganese
- selenium
- zinc

For information on which foods are good sources of these nutrients, *see Chapter 10.*

NAPPY RASH

Nappy rash is common and affects many babies at some time in infancy.

There are four main causes, and it is important to tell them apart so that the right treatment is given:

1. chemical irritation from soiled nappies
2. Candida fungal infection (thrush)
3. bacterial infection
4. allergy to creams, detergents or wipes.

The commonest cause of nappy rash is chemical irritation from soiled nappies and the baby's own waste products. Ammonia forms when bacteria in the faeces break down a chemical, urea, found in the urine. Ammonia is a powerful scouring agent that can easily burn if left on delicate skin for any length of time. Strong intestinal enzymes designed to digest food are also present in baby's bowel motions, as are organic acids made from bacteria fermentation of dietary fibre in the colon. These chemicals can all digest delicate skin in the nappy region, causing soreness, redness and rawness (napkin dermatitis). A nappy rash due to this type of chemical burn usually leaves skin creases unaffected, as chemicals tend not to seep into skin folds. This is a useful way of telling a chemical rash from an infective

(Candida or bacterial) rash. Nappy rashes due to infection tend to involve the skin creases as well, because yeasts and bacteria like creeping into the protection of warm, moist skin folds.

Yeast cells are present on the skin of most young babies and – as the baby's immune system is still immature – will quickly invade the skin if it becomes broken or inflamed. This commonly happens in the nappy area or in skin folds (for example behind the ears, in the armpits).

Thrush causes a red rash with a well-defined edge. The skin tends to be moist and bright red, with scattered spots of infection further away from the main area. These are known as satellite lesions. Unlike the chemical nappy rash, skin folds in the area are usually involved in a thrush rash, too.

Bacterial nappy rashes can be difficult to tell from Candida ones. They are also bright red, may seem to centre around the cleft between the baby's buttocks, and may cause small collections of pus. The baby may seem unwell and may have a fever, in which case you must contact your doctor straightaway. You should also seek immediate medical advice if the nappy rash has open sores, yellow crusts or spots.

SYMPTOMS OF CANDIDA NAPPY RASH

- multiple small red spots in nappy area (these spots may join up to form a more generalized redness of nappy area)
- the rash will involve skin creases, for example at the top of the legs, as well
- red spots (satellite lesions) spread outside the main affected area
- soreness
- blistering and weeping areas
- possibly a build-up of white clots and, occasionally, pustules.

Investigation

If a baby with nappy rash shows signs of being unwell (for example if he has a temperature, is off his feeds or is snuffly or shows other symptoms) it is important to seek medical advice in case a bacterial infection is present. Swabs can be sent for analysis to confirm a yeast infection and rule out a bacterial rash.

Treatment

The treatment of a simple chemical nappy rash is relatively simple:

- Change nappies frequently, as soon as they are soiled.
- If using washable nappies, use an enzyme-free powder and make sure nappies are thoroughly rinsed to remove all traces of detergent.
- Cleanse the nappy area every time you change a nappy – use oil, petroleum jelly or plenty of water, but no soap. Make sure you remove all cream from the previous nappy change to avoid a build-up of waste products and cream.
- Dry the area thoroughly with a tissue or a hair-dryer set on gentle heat.
- Whenever possible, leave the baby's bottom exposed to the air – let your baby lie *on* the nappy rather than *in* it as much as possible, even if only for an hour or two.
- Before putting the baby's nappy on, use large quantities of a barrier cream containing zinc oxide, titanium dioxide, silicone or castor oil. This protects the skin from chemical irritation. Don't use a barrier cream when baby's bottom is exposed to the air, however, as this will prevent the air getting to the skin – only use it when applying a nappy.
- During the night, use a good quality disposable nappy. Choose one that has a one-way layer next to the baby's skin and a built-in plastic backing to help keep skin comfortable and dry.
- If using cloth nappies at any time, use a good quality one-way nappy liner with them.
- Don't use plastic overpants with nappies, as these keep the skin hot and moist.
- If the rash doesn't clear up quickly, ask your doctor or health visitor for advice; an anti-fungal cream or other treatment may be needed.

Treatment of a Candidal nappy rash also involves keeping the affected area clean, dry and exposed to the air as much as possible. You will also need to apply an anti-Candidal cream such as clotrimazole to affected skin 3 times a day. If the skin is very inflamed and raw, a cream combining the anti-fungal with an anti-inflammatory agent (for example 1 per cent hydrocortisone) is often prescribed. Continue using the cream for at least a week after the rash seems to have cleared up, to prevent a recurrence.

A bacterial nappy rash needs urgent treatment with antibiotics to prevent the infection spreading and the baby becoming unwell – if in doubt, consult your health visitor, practice nurse or GP.

Prevention

- Check your baby's nappies frequently so they can be changed as soon as they are soiled.
- Cleanse the skin thoroughly with oil, cream or water (not soap) after each dirty nappy
- Dry thoroughly and apply a protective barrier cream.
- Use a barrier cream before re-applying a nappy.
- If using non-disposable nappies, use a good one-way nappy liner with them.
- Occasionally, a recurrent nappy rash is due to an allergy to chemicals in baby creams, detergents or wipes (for example lanolin, chlorhexidine). If a rash does not respond to normal treatment, or keeps coming back, it is worth trying to avoid perfumed baby products containing plain zinc and castor oil to see if this helps.

ATHLETE'S FOOT

Athlete's foot, or *tinea pedis*, is the most common fungal skin infection affecting as many as 10–15 per cent of the population at any one time. It is highly contagious and is often picked up at communal changing rooms and showers. Fungal spores are also in the air and often lurk in shoes, ready to strike whenever conditions are ripe. It may be triggered by inadequate drying of the spaces between the toes after washing or when skin is rubbed and blistered. Although the toewebs – especially that between the two smallest toes – are usually the first sites to be infected, or ignored and left untreated, the infection can spread to involve the soles and back of the foot as well as the toe- or fingernails themselves. Athlete's foot can be caused by Candida yeasts or dermatophyte infections.

Symptoms

- redness
- build-up of white, dead skin with peeling of skin between the toes (erosio interdigitalis blastomycetica)
- moistness
- itching
- soreness
- formation of painful cracks
- a spreading, dry scaling rash across the surface of the foot
- cracking, brittleness and discoloration of nails.

If an unpleasant smell occurs, this usually means the damaged skin has also become super-infected with bacteria.

Investigation

Investigations are not usually needed for athlete's foot confined to the toeweb unless a secondary bacterial infection is also suspected. Swabs will help to identify the cause. If the nails are affected, nail clippings and skin parings may be sent for analysis to culture and identify the type of fungus present.

Treatment

Don't ignore athlete's foot, as the infection can rapidly spread to involve the nails. Once embedded there treatment will take months and the fungus can be difficult to eradicate. You can also spread infection to elsewhere on your body, for example the hands and nails, through scratching – this can cause the so-called 'Right hand, Left foot' syndrome in right-handed people. Always continue treatment for at least 10 days after symptoms seem to have disappeared, to prevent a recurrence.

If the affected skin area is intact, an anti-fungal powder spray is the easiest treatment to use. This should not be used on broken skin, however, so if cracking has occurred use an anti-fungal cream instead. An anti-fungal powder can also be dusted over the cream and on the foot to keep the skin dry during treatment.

- Benzoyl peroxide/potassium hydroxyquinolone sulphate cream: applied sparingly night and morning
- Clotrimazole cream/powder: 2 or 3 times a day and continued for 2 weeks after symptoms have gone
- Miconazole cream/spray/powder: twice a day and continued for 10 days after healing
- Econazole cream: 2 or 3 times a day and continued for 10 days after healing
- Tolnaftate cream/powder/aerosol: twice a day
- Sulconazole cream (prescription only): massaged in twice a day and used for 2–3 weeks after healing
- Terbinafine cream (prescription only): massaged in once or twice a day for 2–4 weeks
- Amorolfine cream (prescription only): once daily in the evening for 2–3 weeks, continued for 3–5 days after healing
- Nystatin cream/ointment/gel (prescription only): 2–4 times a day until 1 week after healing.

If athlete's foot has spread to the soles of the feet, it will usually only respond to treatment taken by mouth. The skin layer here is much thicker than anywhere else on the body, and it is difficult for treatment creams to penetrate down to the deepest layers. Terbinafine tablets, taken daily for 2 weeks, or itraconazole capsules taken daily for 4 weeks may be prescribed by your doctor.

Prevention

- Take steps to prevent excessive sweating, for example by using an aluminium hexahydrate anti-perspirant (*see page 31*).

- Wash feet every day to remove acidic, sweaty secretions.
- Dry feet thoroughly, especially between the toes – use tissue paper or a hair-dryer set on gentle heat.
- Change socks, stockings or tights at least daily.
- Wear open-toed shoes/sandals as often as possible – avoid wearing synthetic nylon trainers for prolonged periods of time.
- Spray inside shoes and socks with an anti-fungal powder spray, or dust with powder before wearing.
- Discard shoes such as trainers which have developed an unpleasant rotted smell.
- Don't share towels or bath mats.

FUNGAL NAIL INFECTIONS

The nails are specialized skin structures made of a tough protein, keratin. This is secreted by cells at the base and sides of each nail in the matrix. Nails help to strengthen the tips of fingers and toes, protect them from damage and splint the end of the fingers so that the fingertips are more sensitive to touch. The average fingernail grows at a rate of up to 5 mm per month, while the toenails grow 3 times more slowly. It takes around 6 months for a fingernail to grow from base to tip. Nail growth is slower in the non-dominant hand (the left hand if you are right-handed) and slows with increasing age.

Fungal nail infections are known as *tinea unguum* or *onychomycosis*. If the problem is severe with breakdown and distortion of the nail plate, you may be told you have *onycholysis*, in which the nail starts to lift off from its underlying bed. Fungal nail infections are thought to affect up to 3 per cent of the population at any one time. Unfortunately, the condition is often ignored – especially if it only affects hidden toenails – or is disguised by nail varnish. This is not a good idea, as the nails will become riddled with fungal/yeast cells and act as a source of infection that can spread elsewhere on the body, for example to skin folds, the groin, etc. You can also pass the infection on to other members of your family.

Infection of the skin around a nail (*paronychia*) often occurs in people whose work involves repeated wetting of their hands, for example housewives, bar staff, nurses, etc. This leads to redness and swelling of the skin and often a brownish discoloration of one side of the nail. The usual cause of a single infected nail is a bacterial infection, while if many nails are affected (chronic paronychia) the usual cause is a combined *Candida albicans* yeast plus a bacterial infection.

Symptoms

Early symptoms may start as soreness around the edge of the nail (*paronychia*), which spreads to cause:

- thickening of nail folds
- loss of cuticles
- unsightly ridges on the nail
- brittle, flaking, split nails
- dingy discoloration of the nail plate due to infection of the matrix cells which secrete the nail plate
- white patches on the nails (*leukonychia*) – although most white markings are due to mild trauma to the nail bed
- lifting of the nail from its bed (*onycholysis*)
- thickened, distorted nails (*onychogryphosis*).

Investigation

The nails are affected by many illnesses and may develop ridges, pits or discoloration that resemble a fungal infection. For example, a serious illness can produce multiple horizontal ridges, psoriasis can cause roughness and pits, while iron deficiency causes splitting, brittleness, pallor and, if severe, a spoon-like curvature (*koilonychia*). If you develop a nail problem it is important to consult a doctor for a proper diagnosis. If a fungal infection is suspected, nail clippings may be sent for analysis.

Treatment

Paronychia (infection of skin around the nail)
Use a nystatin cream 2–4 times daily. A course of oral antibiotics may be needed if a bacterial infection is also present.

Onychomycosis (infection of the nail itself)

Simple infections can be treated by applying anti-fungal creams or an anti-fungal nail lacquer that hardens to protect the nail as it treats the infection. Alternatively, tablets may be taken by mouth, but prolonged courses are needed.

The damage to the old nail cannot be repaired, and it is difficult to kill the fungal infection riddling it. The aim of treatment is to protect the new nail growing through – so that as your new nail plate develops, it looks pink and healthy compared to the scarred, discoloured nail slowly moving further away from your nail bed.

Treatment should be continued until all the old infected nail has grown through and has been cut and discarded. If treatment is stopped, fungus/yeasts will usually grow down into the new nail from the old infected one and treatment has to be started all over again.

- Amorolfine nail lacquer: applied once or twice a week for 3–6 months
- Tioconazole nail solution: twice a day for 6–12 months
- Terbinafine tablets (prescription only): once a day for 6 weeks – toenail infections require therapy for 3 months
- Itraconazole capsules: once a day for 6 weeks – toenail infections require therapy for 3 months
- Griseofulvin tablets (prescription only): 1–4 times a day. Works well over 6 months' duration for treating fingernail disease, but has a cure rate of only 30–40 per cent for toenail infections, even when treatment is prolonged for 1 year.

Prevention

- Keep nails as dry as possible.
- Use cotton gloves inside rubber ones when washing up or having to put your hands into water.
- Avoid manicures, which can damage cuticles and nail folds – if you wish to have one, make sure it is performed professionally and not by an amateur.
- Avoid using artificial nails.
- Avoid using nail varnish.
- Don't bite or suck your nails.

Chapter Five

CANDIDA INFECTION OF THE GENITALS

MALE GENITALS

Candida infection of the male genitals is common. The groin is a warm, moist, sweaty area that harbours a variety of bacteria and yeasts. In hot conditions – in summer, on holiday abroad or after exercise – Candida yeasts may overgrow to cause symptoms.

Balanitis

Candida yeast infection is the most common problem to affect the tip of the penis. This is known as balanitis and affects up to 5 per cent of young boys, usually striking before school age. Older males can also be affected. Inflammation around the foreskin is called posthitis, and when both occur together – which they frequently do – the result is known as balano-posthitis.

Mild Candidal balanitis may result just in mottled red spots, slight soreness and itching of the tip of the penis. There may also be a build-up of yeasty smegma under the foreskin. If the condition is left untreated and becomes worse, the skin may break down to leave weeping areas, a sticky discharge and painful swelling of the foreskin. This may lead to difficulty passing urine.

Symptoms
- itching on end of penis
- soreness of end of penis
- red spots
- white plaques

- build-up of white material under the foreskin
- pain on passing urine (dysuria).

Other causes of balanitis include infection with common skin bacteria, sexually transmittable diseases, allergic reactions to soap or bath additives and chemical irritation (for example nappy rash in babies).

Investigation
Swabs may be sent for examination to see whether the infection is due to yeasts, bacteria or both. Urinalysis to check for glucose is important to rule out sugar diabetes, in which balanitis is often one of the first signs in men.

Treatment
A study among 43 men with mild balanitis showed that by just washing the penis with water alone, almost all symptoms disappeared without the need for further treatment. It is important not to use soap as this will cause irritation and change skin acidity, making the inflammation and infection worse.

Moderate to severe balanitis due to Candida will need medical assessment to exclude a bacterial infection or overtight foreskin. If a yeast infection is confirmed, treatment is with a topical anti-fungal agent. A cream or gel is less greasy than an ointment and will feel more comfortable. If you are very sore, however, an ointment will provide a barrier that protects skin from contact with urine and stale sweat. You may also find it helpful to use an anti-fungal powder spray around the groin, scrotum and tops of the legs to keep the area clean, dry and prevent the infection spreading under cover of the warmth and humidity of your underpants.

- Clotrimazole cream/spray/powder: applied 2 or 3 times a day and ideally continued for 2 weeks after symptoms have gone, to prevent a recurrence
- Miconazole cream/spray/powder: twice a day and continued for 10 days after healing
- Econazole cream: 2 or 3 times a day and continued for 10 days after healing

- Sulconazole cream (prescription only): massaged in twice a day and used for 2–3 weeks after healing
- Terbinafine cream (prescription only): massaged in once or twice a day for 2–4 weeks
- Amorolfine cream (prescription only): apply once daily in the evening for 2–3 weeks, continuing for 3–5 days after healing
- Nystatin cream/ointment/gel (prescription only): 2–4 times a day until 1 week after healing.

If balanitis is severe, with gross swelling of the foreskin, or if it is recurrent, circumcision may be necessary.

Although Candida is not necessarily sexually transmitted, it is a sexually transmittable disease. It is important to avoid intercourse until symptoms have disappeared, as it is easy to pass the infection on to your partner. Alternatively – assuming your symptoms aren't too unpleasant – you should use a condom together with the spermicide nonoxynol-9, which has some anti-fungal action.

Prevention

Balanitis can largely be prevented by proper hygiene and frequent washing under the foreskin. In mild cases, simple bathing with salt water (saline) twice per day will quickly help symptoms to resolve. Some cases of balanitis are also due to detergent allergy or irritation.

When washing baby boys, the foreskin should never be forcibly retracted – in 96 per cent of babies the foreskin is still attached to the front of the glans penis; forcing it open can cause tissue damage, bleeding and scarring. The natural adhesions break down over the first few years of life – except for the normal attachment underneath, the frenulum – until by the age of 3, 90 per cent of foreskins are partially separated. Tissue remnants may remain up until the age of 17, however.

Males over the age of 7 years who have not been circumcised and whose foreskin can be gently retracted should be taught how to wash underneath the foreskin and should then do so at least once a day – and preferably after every urination. After washing, it is important to make sure the foreskin is pulled forward again to cover the tip of the penis. If it is left back, its blood supply may become restricted leading to swelling (paraphimosis).

Jock-Strap Itch or Dhobie Itch

Candida yeast cells live in the skin creases of up to 80 per cent of the population. They commonly overgrow when conditions are right (that is, warm, moist) to produce an infection around the male groin, scrotum and top of the thighs. This part of your body is often encased in warm, tight-fitting synthetic underwear, tight trousers or sports cloths, which keep conditions hot and humid – ideal for Candida overgrowth.

Other fungi may also be involved and the condition is usually referred to as *tinea cruris* (literally fungal infection of the groin). The first symptom is often itching, followed by the appearance of a dry, red rash with a sharply defined edge. Small pustules may form around hair follicles. If you are prone to heavy sweating in this area, the skin may break down (macerate) to leave raw, weeping areas, especially if you are overweight. The sores ooze a straw-coloured fluid which may harden to form a pale brown crust.

Symptoms
- itching around the scrotum and tops of the legs
- soreness in skin folds
- yeasty, stale-smelling sweat
- red/brown rash with a distinct advancing edge
- sometimes small pustules around hair follicles
- sometimes white plaques
- moist skin breakdown with oozing
- sometimes formation of pale brown crusts
- dark pigmentation of skin
- pain on walking (from the friction of clothes).

Investigation
Swabs may be sent for examination to see whether the infection is due to yeasts, other skin fungi or bacteria. Urinalysis to check for glucose is important to rule out sugar diabetes.

Treatment

Scrupulous hygiene is important to get on top of the infection. You will need to bathe the area regularly with warm water or saline (salt) solution.

Try to keep the area as dry as possible. After washing, pat skin dry with tissue paper or blow dry with a hair-dryer set on gentle heat. Where possible, expose the affected skin to the air as often as possible – for example, wear a long, loose T-shirt with no underpants or trousers when you are home on your own. If this is not possible, wear clothes that are loose and allow air to circulate.

Treatment creams in a vanishing base are less greasy and messy to use during the day when wearing clothes. An ointment will protect sore, weeping areas from crusting and sticking to clothes. An anti-fungal powder spray will help to keep the groin dry.

Treatment preparations are the same as those for treating balanitis (*see page 46*).

Prevention

- Wash the groin area regularly, especially in hot weather and after exercise.
- Dry skin thoroughly after washing.
- Wear loose clothes that allow air to circulate – avoid tight jeans, cycling shorts, etc.
- Wear loose underpants and trousers made from natural fibres rather than man-made ones.
- Choose boxer shorts made from cotton, rather than tight jockey-style briefs.
- After an attack, continue using a dry powder anti-fungal spray to prevent a recurrence.
- Don't share bath towels.

FEMALE GENITALS

The Normal Vulva and Vagina

The vulva is the name for the visible, external female genitalia. It is made up of the clitoris, two outer fleshy folds of skin (labia majora, or large lips) and two smaller, thinner inner folds (labia minora, or small lips). The most common problem affecting this area is itchiness (*pruritis vulvae*). This is usually accompanied by vaginal itching, as well. Vulval itching may be accompanied by redness and soreness, in which case it is known as vulvitis (inflammation of the vulva).

The vagina normally measures around 8 cm (3.25 inches) in length. The corrugated front and back walls are in contact and form an H-shape in cross-section which expands during intercourse and childbirth. During sexual arousal, vaginal tissues become increasingly engorged, changing in colour from rosy pink to purplish red and producing lots more discharge as fluid is forced out of engorged blood vessels under pressure.

Normal Vaginal Discharge

Because the vagina is the most efficient self-cleansing organ in the body, a certain amount of vaginal discharge is both natural and inevitable. A healthy discharge is characterized by being:

- relatively light rather than profuse
- non-irritant
- white or buff in colour
- slightly acidic with a fresh smell that is not offensive.

Your vaginal discharge has a number of important functions, including:

- flushing the vagina clean
- protecting the vaginal lining (epithelial) cells from drying out
- protecting against infection
- preventing chaffing

- providing lubrication during intercourse
- acting as a sexual attractant.

Vaginal discharge contains:
- watery secretions made up of mucus (a glycoprotein made from sugar and protein) and fluid
- sloughed cells from the cervix and vaginal lining (epithelial cells)
- infection-fighting pus cells – these are usually scant but may be profuse when infection is present
- antibodies that help to fight infection
- normal, healthy (commensal) bacteria such as *Lactobacillus*
- potential disease-causing organisms (pathogens) that are normally kept in check by the healthy commensal bacteria
- menstrual debris (blood and endometrial lining cells) during a period
- semen and sperm for a short time after making love without a condom.

How Your Vaginal Discharge Changes throughout the Month

If you are not using a hormonal method of contraception your vaginal discharge will change naturally throughout each monthly cycle. In the first 2 weeks of your cycle (day 1 is the first day of your last period) cervical mucus is mainly under the influence of the female hormone, oestrogen. This keeps it fluid and slippery so that it can be drawn between two fingers to a length of several centimetres. It has an appearance and consistency similar to raw egg white. This thin cervical mucus is sperm-friendly. Its molecules are all lined up in a similar direction and sperm can swim through it easily and survive in it for a relatively long time.

Immediately after ovulation, cervical mucus comes under the influence of progesterone hormone and suddenly changes virtually overnight to become scant, thick and sticky. Its molecules become entangled, rather like barbed wire, so that the mucus becomes hostile to sperm – they cannot swim through easily and perish quickly. These changes in the quantity, fluidity, glossiness, transparency and elasticity of vaginal secretions are monitored regularly by women using the natural, fertility awareness method of contraception.

Vulvo-Vaginal Candidiasis

Candida infection is the most common cause of inflammation of the vagina (vaginitis) and the outer surrounding area (vulvitis). If it affects both sites simultaneously, it is known as vulvo-vaginitis.

Candida is found normally as a harmless (commensal) organism in the vagina of many women without causing symptoms. When vaginal swabs are taken and grown in special cultures which encourage the overgrowth of Candida cells, yeasts are detected in 10–55 per cent of apparently well women (the average seems to be 1 in 5, or 20 per cent) who have no symptoms of thrush infection at all. In these cases, yeast cells are either present in an inactive state (as resting spores) or surviving quite happily in low numbers, kept in check by other healthy bacteria such as *Lactobacillus acidophilus*. During the symptomless phase, active yeasts are present as simple cells (non-filamentous forms) in relatively small numbers rather than in the filamentous form with hyphae (yeast cell germ tubes – *see page 2*).

Whether the yeast cells come and go or are present all the time is not really known. Studies suggest that Candida remains in the vagina for at least several months, and possibly for years at a time without causing obvious harm. If the natural balance is tipped, however – due to changing levels of hormones, acidity, sugar content or the numbers and types of bacteria present – Candida cells may suddenly proliferate to cause symptoms which may include:

- itching
- redness
- soreness
- vaginal dryness
- a white, cottage-cheese-like discharge
- a yeasty smell
- pain on intercourse
- cystitis-like pain on passing urine (dysuria)
- increased frequency of urination
- enlarged, tender lymph nodes (glands) in the groin.

The amount of discharge does not necessarily relate to the severity of symptoms, and some women find that vaginal dryness makes their other symptoms worse.

Other causes of itching and soreness which may be confused with Candida include:

- other infections, such as anaerobic vaginosis, Herpes simplex (cold sore) virus, Human papilloma (wart) virus
- allergy to chemicals in deodorants, spermicides, creams, douches, bath products, soaps, lubricants and, rarely, to sperm and semen themselves
- lack of oestrogen after the menopause (atrophic vulvo-vaginitis)
- skin changes linked with ageing (vulval dystrophies)
- chemical irritation due to urinary leakage (as caused, for example, by stress incontinence).

Simple itching may also be caused by infections such as pubic lice and scabies, or skin problems such as eczema or psoriasis which can affect this area as well as other parts of the body.

Vaginal Acidity and Candida

The acidity of vaginal secretions changes throughout your menstrual cycle. For most of the month, secretions are acidic. This partly results from acids secreted by your own vaginal cells, but most are made by friendly bacteria such as *Lactobacillus acidophilus* as a by-product of their metabolism. These 'gold-standard' bacteria thrive in acid conditions and usually keep Candida infections at bay by competing with them for micronutrients, food (glycogen/glucose) and binding sites which both organisms (Lactobacilli and Candida) use to stick to the epithelial cells in your vaginal walls.

As your period approaches, natural hormone changes mean that your vaginal discharge becomes less acidic. Blood itself is slightly alkaline, and during menstruation this makes the vaginal environment much less acid again. This affects the friendly bacteria present in your vagina. They struggle due to lack of acidity, which means it is easier for Candida to take over and proliferate.

When conditions are acidic, Candida tends to stay in its less invasive form as simple yeasts cells. When conditions become less acid and near neutral, Candida tends to produce threads (germ tubes, or hyphae) which are more invasive and likely to trigger symptoms. This switch from a simple-celled form to the thread form occurs at around pH 6 (just below neutral) and can happen within 1 to 3 hours of a change in environmental conditions. As a result, vaginal Candidiasis is more common around the time of your period.

Sugar Content of Vaginal Discharge and Candida

During the second half of your menstrual cycle (after ovulation) hormone changes increase the glycogen content of vaginal cells. Glycogen is a starchy storage compound that is broken down in the cells to provide sugar (glucose) as an energy source – it is also a favourite fuel for developing yeast cells.

With the tailing off of acidity that also occurs around the time of a period, increased cell sugar content increases the risk of developing thrush. Women with sugar diabetes (*Diabetes mellitus*) also have increased sugar levels in their vaginal secretions unless their condition is tightly controlled by diet, insulin injections or sugar-lowering drugs. This increases the risk of Candidal vulvo-vaginitis, and many new cases of diabetes are picked up each year when women with recurrent Candida are routinely screened for the presence of excess sugar in the urine or blood.

Synthetic Hormones and Vulvo-vaginal Candida

Many women who have problems with vaginal discharge and Candida are on the contraceptive Pill or taking certain types of hormone replacement therapy (HRT). Synthetic hormones alter the normal monthly changes that occur in the vaginal discharge cycle, and can change normal vaginal acidity. Your discharge may become continuously thin and watery or thick and barely there, depending on which blend of combined oral contraceptive Pill or HRT you are using.

Hormone treatments that are predominantly oestrogenic (contain more oestrogen compared with progestogen) encourage increased vaginal secretions which tend to be thin, elastic and sometimes copious. This is partly because they increase the number of mucus-secreting cells found around the cervix. Oestrogen also seems to increase the stickiness of vaginal cells, so that Candida yeasts are more likely to bind to them. It also stimulates production of a yeast-fibre network (mycelium) so that it spreads more quickly. Hormone treatments that are relatively progestogenic (contain more progestogen compared with oestrogen) produce the opposite effect – scant, thick mucus which is accompanied by vaginal dryness.

Taking synthetic hormones can also affect the glycogen/sugar content of vaginal cells, so that women taking the oral contraceptive Pill or HRT also seem to be at increased risk of developing vulvo-vaginal Candida. This is most likely if the hormone blend you are on contains relatively high doses of oestrogen. Blends containing low doses of oestrogen are less likely to cause problems with vulval or vaginal thrush.

Pregnancy and Vulvo-vaginal Candida

During pregnancy, vulvo-vaginal thrush is so common that 30–40 per cent of women develop symptoms at least once during their pregnancy.

- Pregnancy is a time when the mother's natural immunity is lowered so that the developing baby, who contains 'foreign' genes inherited from the father, is not attacked by the mother's defences.
- Very high levels of circulating hormones increase the glycogen/sugar content of vaginal cells – pregnancy is also a time when the body's ability to metabolize sugar becomes increasingly impaired, so that sugar levels throughout the body are likely to be higher than normal. This provides increased carbohydrate to fuel the growth and division of Candida cells.
- High levels of oestrogen (as found in pregnancy) seem to increase the stickiness of vaginal cells so that Candida yeasts are more likely to bind to them – oestrogen also seems to

stimulate the production of the yeast's fibre network so that it spreads more quickly.

- During pregnancy, high levels of progesterone are produced. This hormone has a relaxant effect on smooth muscle cells throughout the body, so that the vagina may not flush its secretions through as effectively as normal.
- Increased needs to visit the bathroom due to pressure of the growing womb on the bladder and bowel increase the risk of gut Candida being transferred from the bowel to the vagina.

Thrush is most likely to strike during the last 3 months of pregnancy, and recurrences are common. Unfortunately, it also seems that standard treatments are less effective during pregnancy – presumably because the Candida have so many positive environmental factors in their favour that they can survive a certain exposure to anti-fungal agents.

Antibiotics and Vulvo-vaginal Candida

Many women notice that their symptoms develop during or after a course of antibiotics. The most common culprits are so-called broad-spectrum antibiotics (for example tetracycline, ampicillin, amoxycillin, cephalosporins) which wipe out some of the healthy bacteria found in the vagina as well as the disease-causing bugs they are designed to treat. These healthy bacteria (especially *Lactobacillus*) keep Candida at bay by competing with it for nutrients and for binding sites to vaginal lining cells and by secreting chemicals that increase the acidity of the environment and inhibit yeast cell growth. When women on antibiotics are screened for the presence of vaginal Candida (even if they are not having any symptoms), yeast cells are found in 3 times more women than among a similar group not on antibiotics. Thrush spores are present in the air and germinate in warm, moist places. Candida thrives when natural immunity falls, as during times of stress and illness or when antibiotics destroy the normal vaginal bacteria that keep yeast infections at bay.

Lack of Iron and Vulvo-vaginal Candida

White blood cells need the mineral iron to make an array of powerful chemicals used to combat infections such as Candida. Even a mild iron deficiency can result in reduced immunity – although the deficiency may not be pronounced enough to cause anaemia. While your blood count (haemoglobin concentration) may be normal, a low reserve of iron can be detected by measuring blood levels of an iron compound called ferritin. Ferritin is the main way iron is stored in the body and one of the ways it is transported around the circulation. It is made up of a protein, apoferritin, linked to a varying number of iron atoms – one molecule of apoferritin may contain as many as 4,500 atoms of iron. When iron stores are low, less apoferritin is made, and iron in the bloodstream moves from apoferritin to another iron-transporting protein, transferrin.

Ideally, all women suffering from recurrent thrush should have their ferritin level measured. If it is low, treatment with an iron-containing vitamin and mineral supplement may be enough to solve the problem, although this remedy will need to be continued for several months until iron stores are back to normal. If you are found to have a low ferritin level, you and your doctor will also need to think about why your iron levels are low:

- Do you eat a good, nutritious diet full of iron-rich foods? (*see page 155*)
- Do you suffer from heavy or frequent periods?
- Have your iron stores been depleted through pregnancy?
- Are you losing hidden blood from your bowels?
- Does your body have a problem absorbing the iron in your diet?
- Is there a problem with production of red blood cells in your marrow?

If the iron deficiency is significant, you may well need investigations to find out its cause.

WHERE IRON IS FOUND IN THE BODY

- 70 per cent of body iron is in the red blood pigment, haemoglobin
- 3 per cent is in the red muscle pigment, myoglobin
- 27 per cent is in the form of ferritin

Tight Synthetic Clothes and Vulvo-vaginal Candida

Wearing tight or poorly ventilated underclothes – especially those fashioned from man-made fibres that are unable to 'breathe' – are strongly linked with an increased risk of developing vulvo-vaginal Candida. This is because yeast spores love to germinate in warm, moist places; tight clothes increase the humidity and temperature of vulval skin creases. If you suffer from recurrent vaginal thrush, it may be helpful to wear loose, well-ventilated clothes and cotton underwear. Avoid nylon tights, and instead wear stockings – either those with elasticated tops that stay up on their own, or with a suspender belt for support.

Low-Temperature Wash Cycles and Candida

In the old days, underwear was given a thorough, regular boil-up in a pan of water on top of the stove. Modern wash-day practices often involve the use of low-temperature wash cycles to protect delicate fashion lingerie. As a result, Candida spores may survive the process and linger in your underwear, to cause reinfection. There are several ways in which you can prevent this:

- Continue washing your lingerie as before, but iron the cotton gussets with a very hot iron to kill any residual Candida spores.
- Pre-soak underwear in concentrated detergent and scrub the crotch before putting them into the wash.
- Wear white cotton underwear, which can survive a hot wash without undue damage
- Soak pants in bleach (if the material will take it) before washing.

Don't, however, put your underpants in the microwave as was once recommended – they may go up in smoke!

These simple measures are often enough to break the misery of recurrent thrush infection.

Sun Beds and Candida

Some women seem to suffer a bout of Candida after using a sun bed. This is partly due to the increased warmth and moistness generated while under the lamps. Ultra-violet light is known to trigger recurrences of Herpes simplex infection, and it has recently been discovered that Candida can 'switch' (*see page 14*) from their smooth form to a rough one when exposed to low doses of ultraviolet light. The switched (rough) colonies produce different patterns of germ tube threads (hyphae) and seem to:

- proliferate more readily
- stick to body lining cells more easily, making it easier to invade tissues
- secrete more enzymes that break down proteins, fats and cell walls
- be more invasive
- escape from detection by immune cells more easily
- be less susceptible to anti-fungal treatments.

Using a sun bed may therefore trigger symptoms of thrush in someone who has previously lived quite happily with Candida without developing symptoms.

While washing the vulval area after using a sun bed and wearing loose cotton clothes may help to prevent an attack of thrush due to increased humidity and warmth, it is worth avoiding sun beds altogether if you suffer from recurrent Candidiasis.

Investigation

While your doctor may suspect a diagnosis of vulval or vaginal thrush just by asking you questions about your symptoms, it is important that you are examined and a swab taken to confirm the diagnosis. If the infection is advanced, the vagina may be full of thick, white cottage-cheese-like clots that are obviously due to a yeast infection. In mild or early cases, however, the mucous membranes may just look red and there may be a grey-white-yellow discharge similar to that seen in other common vaginal conditions such as:

- Gardnerella vaginalis
- Bacterial vaginosis (anaerobic bacterial imbalance)
- Herpes simplex infection
- Trichomonas vaginalis
- Chlamydia
- Early wart virus infection (itching)
- Pubic lice (itching)
- Skin problems such as eczema or psoriasis.

Don't be afraid to ask for an examination and for a swab to be sent to hospital. Similarly, if you decide to treat your symptoms of vulvo-vaginal Candida yourself with over-the-counter products, always consult your doctor if the symptoms don't start to clear up quickly (within 3–5 days).

Sending vaginal swabs to hospital for culture is not always helpful, as delays in transit may mean that Candida cells in the swab may die and go undetected. If you continue to have problems of vulvo-vaginal irritation, soreness or discharge but swabs persistently claim to be negative or normal, don't be embarrassed about attending a genito-urinary medicine (GUM, VD, STD or Special) clinic. You will be treated sympathetically and confidentially and, as fresh secretions are examined under the microscope there and then, any infection is usually picked up quickly. You will also be screened for an infection called chlamydia, which is not usually done in general practice. Chlamydia are too small to be seen under the light microscope and they are extremely difficult to culture. They can only be detected in a cervical swab by using a special immunological technique which takes several days. All genito-urinary clinics will check for this disease, while only a few GPs have the special culture bottle required.

As a bonus, treatments provided by a genito-urinary medicine clinic are free as they do not attract a prescription charge.

A genito-urinary check-up is especially important if you notice:

- any abnormality of your vaginal discharge, for example increased quantity, unusual smell or staining
- itching, soreness, tenderness or pain
- abnormal bleeding
- lumps or ulceration
- pain on urinating (dysuria, cystitis)
- low abdominal pain
- discomfort during intercourse
- genital problems in your sexual partner
- if you are at risk of having contracted a sexually transmittable disease.

Treatment

A number of orthodox treatments are available for treating vulvo-vaginal thrush. Some of these treatments (for example clotrimazole, fluconazole) are now available over the counter, while others remain prescription only. As the situation is constantly changing, with more and more drugs coming off prescription each year, it is worth asking your pharmacist for advice on which treatment will suit you best if you wish to self-medicate:

Clotrimazole:
- 1 per cent cream for use on vulva – applied 2 or 3 times a day and ideally continued for 1 week after symptoms have gone
- pessaries for insertion in the vagina at night:
- 100-mg pessaries are used for 6 nights in a row
- 200-mg pessaries are used for 3 nights in a row
- 500-mg pessary has only to be used for 1 night
- 10 per cent vaginal cream in pre-filled applicator: to be squirted into the vagina last thing at night as a single dose
- 2 per cent vaginal cream plus 6 applicators: squirted into vagina twice a day for 3 days, or used nightly for 6 nights in a row

Econazole:

- 1 per cent cream/lotion: applied 2 or 3 times a day and continued for 1 week after symptoms have gone
- 150-mg long-acting pessary: inserted into vagina at night as a single dose
- 150-mg pessaries: inserted into vagina for 3 nights in a row

Miconazole:

- 2 per cent cream with applicators: inserted into vagina twice a day for 7 days, or used on vulva twice a day
- vaginal capsules (1,200 mg) plus finger stall: inserted into vagina at night as a single dose
- 100-mg pessaries: inserted into vagina twice a day for 7 days

Fenticonazole:

- 200-mg gelatin pessaries: inserted into vagina for 3 nights in a row
- 600-mg gelatin pessary: inserted into vagina at night as a single dose
- Isoconazole: 2 300-mg vaginal tablets inserted into the vagina for a single night

Nystatin:

- cream/gel: applied to vulva 2–4 times a day for 2 weeks
- vaginal cream plus applicators: inserted into vagina for 14 nights in a row
- oral tablets (500,000 units): 4 times a day during vaginal treatment to eradicate gut infection
- Fluconazole: 150-mg capsule taken by mouth as a single dose
- Itraconazole: 2 100-mg capsules taken twice daily for 1 day (total of 4 capsules)
- Ketoconazole: tablets/suspension for oral use in chronic, recurrent vaginal thrush that does not respond to other treatments. Taken once a day with meals for 5 days.

For alternative (complementary health) treatments, see Chapter 9.

Prevention

Self-help remedies to help treat/prevent vulvo-vaginal thrush include:

- Avoid wearing tight underwear, especially nylon pantyhose or tight trousers. Stockings and cotton underwear are best as they allow air to circulate, so that warmth and humidity are reduced.
- Avoid getting hot and sweaty – use panty-liners and change them as necessary throughout the day; shower, wash or bathe immediately after exercise.
- Don't use bath additives, vaginal deodorants or douches – they can upset your natural acid and bacterial balance.
- Avoid trauma to vaginal tissues from vigorous sex or rubbing too hard with a bath towel.
- Try boiling cotton underwear or hot-ironing panty gussets. Modern low-temperature washing machine cycles don't kill Candida spores.
- Use an acid gel (0.9 per cent acetic acid in a jelly base, available over the counter) to help maintain vaginal acidity so that Candida cells remain in their simple non-invasive form.
- Smear the vulva and lower vagina with natural BIO yoghurt containing live *Lactobacillus acidophilus* – these bacteria can colonize the vagina and help to prevent Candida overgrowth. Taking Acidophilus tablets (from healthfood shops), eating BIO yoghurt and drinking Yakult (a culture of *Lactobacillus casei* Shirota) may also help to reduce bowel colonization with thrush (*see page 97*).
- Try following an anti-yeast diet or a simpler regime of cutting out alcohol, mushrooms, sugary foods, tea, coffee and chocolate. Eat a wholefood diet of salads, fruit, vegetables, pulses and wholegrain cereals instead.
- Try to avoid stress – make time for regular exercise, rest and relaxation.
- Take a good multivitamin and mineral supplement containing around 100 per cent of the recommended daily amount (RDA) of as many vitamins and minerals as possible.
- If you are being treated for Candida, make sure your partner

uses an anti-thrush cream too. Thrush spores can survive under the male foreskin without causing any symptoms. They may then be passed back to you.

■ If the problem is recurrent, have a vaginal health check at your local genito-urinary medicine clinic.

Chapter Six

CANDIDA INFECTION OF THE DIGESTIVE TRACT

NORMAL DIGESTION

The intestinal tract is one of the main sites where yeast cells are normally found colonizing the body. In order to understand the problems this may cause, it is worth having a quick look at the normal structure and function of the intestines.

The gastro-intestinal tract is a long tube which starts at the mouth and ends at the anal sphincter. It is basically a food-processing system that accepts complex food molecules at one end and breaks these down into simpler, soluble nutrients which are absorbed into the bloodstream. Waste products are disposed of – usually in neat packages – at the other end.

The Mouth

Digestion starts in the mouth. Saliva contains an enzyme, amylase, which starts breaking down starchy complex carbohydrates into simpler sugars. The teeth chew and grind food into small pieces which are moistened with saliva. Each mouthful is then rolled into a small ball (bolus) by the tongue and pushed to the back of the mouth where it is swallowed by a reflex action. Yeast cells present in your food can easily survive this process.

The Oesophagus and Stomach

The food bolus travels down your gullet (oesophagus) to the stomach, where it is mixed with powerful secretions containing hydrochloric acid and enzymes. Proteins, fats and carbohydrates are broken down into simpler units while muscular contractions

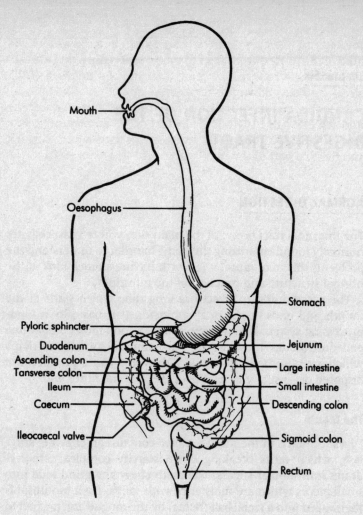

The digestive tract

churn the whole stomach contents to mix the food and digestive juices thoroughly. Food usually spends around 6 hours in your stomach while it is processed and converted into a liquid porridge-like slurry known as chyme.

Glands in your stomach produce around 3 litres of acidic fluid per day. While yeast cells can live quite happily in your mouth and oesophagus, most are usually rapidly killed once they reach your stomach, as long as it is functioning properly. A few will survive the process from time to time – especially if you are taking antacids, which reduce stomach acidity, or have a stomach ulcer – and pass down further into the gut.

Once the food in your stomach is converted into chyme, the stomach exit valve (pyloric sphincter) opens momentarily for a few seconds at a time to let stomach contents squirt through into the first part of the small intestines.

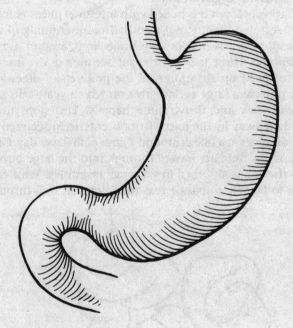

The oesophagus and stomach

The Small Intestines

The small intestines, or foregut, are highly coiled to fit into the abdominal cavity. They form a tube around 285 cm long and 3.5 cm in diameter. The first part of the small intestine after the stomach is the duodenum. The intestinal juices secreted into the duodenum are alkaline, to neutralize acidity from the stomach. Bile from the liver and powerful enzymes from the pancreas also flow into the duodenum to start the next phase of digestion.

The jejunum is the name given to the first 40 per cent of the small intestine below the duodenum, while the next 60 per cent of the small intestine is known as the ileum. As there is no distinct border between the two this division is somewhat arbitrary. Surprisingly, Candida cells can survive quite happily throughout the small intestines, becoming more and more frequent towards the large intestines.

As food travels down it is mixed with intestinal juices (succus entericus) secreted by mucosal glands. The inner lining of the small intestines is covered in tiny projections around 1 mm long, called villi. These increase the surface area of the intestinal wall to speed up absorption of the products of digestion. They also provide a large surface area on which yeast cells and bacteria can stick and thrive quite happily. This stops them being washed away by the juices (succus entericus) secreted by the small intestines at a rate of around 7 litres of fluid per day. Only 1–2 litres of this fluid are passed through into the large bowel, however, the rest is absorbed in the small intestines. Yeast cells also seem to be able to pass across the intestinal wall through

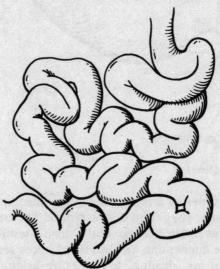

The small intestines

this large surface area of your small intestines in a process known as translocation (*see page 14*). By the time food has reached the end of the small intestines and passed into the large bowel, the process of digestion is complete.

The Large Intestines

The large intestines form a wide tube that is around 1 m long. The large bowel – made up of the colon, rectum and anal canal – is the main site where yeast cells thrive happily in the normal gut. The large intestines are where excess fluid, salts and minerals are absorbed from the gut, while waste – mainly indigestible fibre – is compacted and made ready for an orderly disposal through the anus.

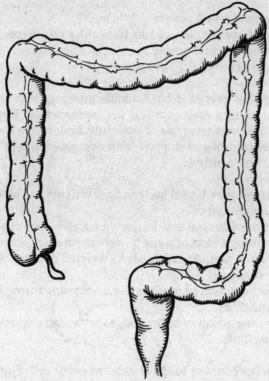

The large intestines

The large intestines are home to billions of bacteria which ferment indigestible fibre waste to produce acids and gases, as well as many useful vitamins such as biotin. Altogether, bowel micro-organisms – including yeasts – make up around 30 per cent of normal stool bulk.

CANDIDA IN THE HEALTHY GUT

The intestinal tract is one of the main sites where yeast cells are normally found colonizing the body. Organisms living in the body in this harmless way are known as *commensals*. When swabs are taken from healthy people, Candida can be grown from:

- the mouth of 1 in 2 people
- the oesophagus (gullet) of 1 in 10 healthy volunteers
- the rectum of 1 in 3 people
- the faeces of 8 out of 10 people

It is likely that everyone has Candida growing in their gut at some time during each year – if not permanently. The gut is thought to act as a reservoir of yeast infection, which is usually kept under control and stopped from overgrowing by a variety of factors. These include:

- competition with bowel bacteria for nutrients and binding sites on intestinal cells
- production of natural anti-fungal chemicals by bowel bacteria
- the sterilizing action of some bowel enzymes and juices
- the action of antibodies (type IgA) secreted onto the inner surface of the gut
- the flushing action of food and liquids passing through the small intestines
- the scouring action of bulky roughage passing through the large intestines.

Yeast cells have to stick to the membrane of the cells lining your gut if they are to survive without being flushed through your system and out the other end. They need to stick to special binding sites on your cell membranes – but these sites are also used by other bowel organisms such as the *Lactobacillus* bacteria. Many healthy bacteria also secrete substances that interfere with the growth of other organisms. Acting together, these different factors usually damp down Candida growth so that it lives quite happily inside you – and may even do you some good. Vitamins made by yeast cells – especially the B group and biotin – seep into your intestinal juices and are readily absorbed.

How Candida Gets into Your Gut

Candida yeasts mostly enter your gut through your mouth:

- in the food that you eat
- from the skin of your hands
- if you suck on anything (pens, etc.) that may have yeast cells on it
- through kissing and oral sex.

Live Candida yeasts are frequently present in food and drinks. In one study which analysed a range of common foods, live Candida cells were recovered from a number of them, of which the worst culprits were:

- fruit juices
- drinks
- ice cubes
- salads
- snacks
- cereals.

With the juices, all vegetable and fruit varieties were affected, including apple, pineapple, orange, tomato, grape, apricot and lemonade. The yeast contamination seemed to be related to the type of packaging and processing used during preparation rather than the type of fruit involved. All juices sealed with foil wraps were contaminated, while those in cans or bottles were yeast-free:

Type of Food	Number of samples tested	Number positive for live Candida yeasts	per cent
Drinks	16	4	25
Breads	8	0	0
Cereals	17	2	12
Condiments	23	0	0
Desserts	39	1	3
Fish	4	0	0
Fruits	6	0	0
Juices	61	38	62
Meats (cooked)	20	0	0
Milk and dairy products	27	1	4
Salads	8	3	38
Sauces	10	0	0
Snacks	25	3	12
Soups	16	0	0
Vegetables	44	2	5
Ready-cooked meals	21	0	0

CANDIDA INFECTION OF THE MOUTH

Candida infection of the mouth (oral thrush) is common. It can occur at any age, but is most often seen in young babies up to the age of 18 months, the middle-aged, and the elderly.

Yeast cells seem to prefer living in certain sites in the mouth more than others. In order of preference, these include:

- upper surface of your tongue
- palate
- inner surfaces of the cheeks
- on dentures, especially upper ones.

Bacteria and yeasts can often be seen on top of the tongue as a white/yellow thick coating which may smell offensive and contribute to bad breath (halitosis).

Mouth infections, including thrush, are more common if you suffer from:

- a dry mouth (zerostomia), which may be due to increasing age, poor saliva production, taking certain drugs (for example, some antihistamines) or prolonged mouth breathing
- asthma and use inhaled corticosteroids to control the underlying inflammation
- diabetes – especially if you also smoke, which seems to lower your resistance to oral thrush
- impaired immunity through illness, stress, drugs or a nutrient deficiency.

People who wear dentures are also more likely to develop oral thrush – known as denture stomatitis. Experiments show that Candida yeasts can stick to the denture material and act as a continuous source of reinfection.

Symptoms

The symptoms of oral thrush may include:

- a thick coating on the tongue
- a red, sore, shiny tongue
- sores at the corners of the lips (angular stomatitis)
- white plaques on the inside of your cheeks
- itching, for example on the roof of your mouth, beneath dentures
- soreness
- dryness (xerostomia)
- pain on eating or drinking
- ulceration inside the mouth.

When oral thrush develops as cream/white curd-like plaques in the mouth, this is known as acute (recent onset) pseudomembranous (false-membrane) Candidiasis. The plaques are easily rubbed away and contain yeast cells, hyphae (yeast cell germ tubes), inflammatory cells, bacteria, lining (epithelial) cells from the mouth, food debris and dead cells which are starting to break down. Underneath the plaque is a raw, tender area that is usually painful and red and which may bleed.

When the plaques are dislodged (for example while you are eating) they leave behind a shiny, red, glossy area that is known as acute (recent onset) atrophic (wasted) Candidiasis. These areas of the tongue usually reveal a localized loss of tastebuds. If left untreated, the lesions take on a lumpy, granular appearance as underlying cells and blood vessels multiply in an attempt to heal small areas of ulceration. This is usually diagnosed as chronic (long-term) atrophic (wasted) Candidiasis.

If still left untreated, these areas may thicken and develop tough, white membranes with a roughened surface. These tend to be larger than the false membranes seen in early thrush infections and cannot be scraped away easily or dislodged during eating. This stage of oral thrush is known as chronic (long-term) hyperplastic (thickened) Candidiasis, or Candidal leukoplakia (white patches). If this type of white patch forms in the mouth, it is important that it is biopsied and properly diagnosed. Other conditions – some of which are precancerous – can also cause white patches (leukoplakia) in the mouth; these need to be picked up early and treated to prevent mouth cancer (*see page 77*).

Investigation

Oral thrush can usually be diagnosed by looking in the mouth and seeing characteristic areas of redness and white patches. Swabs can be examined under the microscope for yeast cells, hyphae and spores, or sent to be cultured in the laboratory to confirm the diagnosis and rule out other causes.

Treatment

Oral thrush is usually easily treated with anti-fungal agents. If you are pregnant or breastfeeding, don't use any preparations before checking with a pharmacist or doctor:

- Mild infections may respond to a Hexetidine antiseptic mouthwash/gargle used 2 or 3 times a day.
- Miconazole gel is available from pharmacies and comes in a pleasant orange-flavoured base. This is used 2–4 times per

day (depending on age). The gel should be held in the mouth for as long as possible before swallowing. It can also be applied directly to lesions using a clean finger. Treatment should be continued for at least 2 days after symptoms have disappeared.

- Sugar-free pastilles containing dequalinium chloride can be bought from pharmacies: to be sucked every 4 hours. They help to treat both bacterial and fungal infections of the mouth and throat.
- Amphotericin lozenges (prescription only): to be sucked 4–8 times daily for up to 15 days. If preferred, an amphotericin suspension can also be inserted into the mouth with a dropper and used 4 times a day for 14 days. Keep both preparations in contact with lesions for as long as possible. Use for at least 2 days after symptoms have disappeared.
- Nystatin pastilles (prescription only): to be sucked 4 times daily – do not eat or drink for 5 minutes before or 1 hour after treatment. If preferred, a suspension for inserting into the mouth with a dropper is also available. Hold preparations against the lesions for as long as possible. Continue for at least 2 days after symptoms have disappeared.

    For severe infections:
- a course of anti-fungal Fluconazole (capsules or suspension) can be prescribed: to be taken once a day for 7–14 days
- a course of Itraconazole (capsules) can be prescribed for use once a day for 15 days (twice a day for patients with an underlying disease affecting their immunity).

If your mouth is really sore, a local anaesthetic spray (for example benzocaine) or anti-inflammatory spray/rinse (for example benzydamine) can be used to help numb the pain.

If you suffer from oral thrush and use dentures, these can be treated using a miconazole denture lacquer which comes in a pack containing 3 bottles, brushes and tissues (prescription only). The entire contents of 1 bottle is applied to the upper surface of a clean, disinfected and dried upper denture. Allow to dry for at least 1 hour before inserting into the mouth. This is repeated twice more at weekly intervals.

Prevention

A mouthwash containing chlorhexidine has some anti-Candida action and may help to keep recurrent oral thrush at bay – but check with your dentist that this will suit you first. Not all dentists recommend chlorhexidine mouthwashes, and they can cause staining of teeth with prolonged use.

If you suffer from a dry mouth, an artificial saliva solution (for example carboxymethyl-cellulose aerosol/spray or mucin xylitol spray) will help to keep your mouth moist and discourage infection. This comes in natural, lemon or peppermint flavours. A pastille containing malic acid can also be sucked to stimulate the flow of saliva.

If you wear dentures, it is important to keep these scrupulously clean and not let stains build up. They should be kept in a sterilizing solution at night and checked regularly by your dentist for signs of wear or infection, and to check their fit.

Most people with asthma need to use a corticosteroid inhaler regularly to damp down the inflammation in their lungs. Even when inhaled correctly, up to 90 per cent of the medication will be deposited in the upper airways and then swallowed – only around 10 per cent of the dose reaches the lungs. As the corticosteroid works by damping down excessive immune reactions in the tissues it touches, this makes oral thrush more likely. It's therefore a good idea to clean your teeth, use a mouthwash or gargle immediately after using your inhaler (especially if it is a dry powder inhaler) to remove remaining particles. If recurrent oral thrush is a problem, ask your doctor about using a device such as a spacer to help minimize the amount of drug that deposits in your throat.

People with gum disease are 4 times more likely to develop a thrush infection than other people. If you have redness or swelling of the gums round your teeth, or if your gums bleed when brushing, you may well have gingivitis (infected gums) which harbour bacteria and yeasts in infected pockets between your gums and teeth. If this is ignored, infection will spread to involve the jawbone round your teeth (periodontitis), and your gums will start to recede. Ignore periodontitis and you will eventually lose your teeth altogether.

Unfortunately, cleaning your teeth twice a day is not enough to solve gum disease. What you need is an expert assessment of your mouth by a dentist committed to oral hygiene, followed by a course of treatment with a dental hygienist. By having your gum pockets cleared of infected plaque and rotting food, gum disease can be beaten. You will then need to continue with a regular programme of proper brushing and flossing, to keep your mouth healthy and disease-free.

Sores at the corners of the mouth where the lips meet (angular stomatitis) are sometimes signs of iron-deficiency anaemia. If you feel tired and washed out, or if the problem is recurrent, it is important to ask your doctor if you might be suffering from anaemia. If so, the cause of this will need to be investigated.

If you smoke, try to stop – smoking damages the lining of your mouth, increases the risk of oral thrush and is also linked with mouth cancer.

Mouth Cancer

Mouth cancer is becoming increasingly common. Around 2,000 new cases are diagnosed each year and it now makes up 5 per cent of all tumours. While mouth cancer is not especially linked with Candida infection, it can be triggered by long-term infections (sepsis) of the mouth or ill-fitting infected dentures. It can be mistaken for chronic hyperplastic Candidiasis. Sadly, the outlook is often poor as mouth cancers have often grown quite large before they are picked up. Those that develop on the roof of the mouth or top of the tongue may be spotted early, but those on the floor of the mouth, under the tongue or in 'coffin corner' – an aptly nick-named crevice lurking at the back of your throat – are difficult to detect in the early stages. Two out of every three sufferers are male, and most cases occur in the over-forties.

Mouth cancer is linked with several risk factors, known as the 5 S's:

1. *Smoking* – those who smoke cigars, a pipe or cigarettes, chew tobacco or inhale snuff are at greatest risk
2. *Spirits* – drinking excessive amounts of alcoholic spirits can trigger oral cancer

3. *Spices* – long-term exposure to hot spices has been linked with this disease
4. *Syphilis* – though this infection is now relatively rare
5. *Sepsis* – chronic irritation or infection from ill-fitting dentures, a jagged tooth or infected gums.

Mouth cancers usually start as a whitish patch (leukoplakia) or a red velvety patch (erythroplakia), both of which can mimic Candida infections. These pre-cancerous changes may cause a slight burning sensation in the mouth, but most are painless. As the tumour develops it will form a small, raised lump which eventually ulcerates or forms a deep crack. This may bleed as it eats into surrounding tissues and is usually quite painful. It is important that you do not continue to treat a mouth lesion which does not respond to anti-thrush treatment for longer than a week or two without consulting a doctor or dentist.

EXAMINING YOUR MOUTH

Most mouth cancers, and many thrush infections, are detected by dentists – an excellent reason to have regular dental check-ups, even if your teeth are perfect. It is also worth inspecting the inside of your mouth yourself from time to time – especially if you're over 40. Use a dental mirror to view the floor of your mouth, underneath and along the sides of your tongue, and the gutters around your gums. The things to look for are:

- unexplained white patches
- unexplained red velvety patches
- raised lumps
- an ulcer that refuses to heal.

Any unexplained mouth ulcer lasting longer than 3 weeks needs full investigation. Similarly, don't ignore a persistent sore throat or hoarseness lasting longer than 3 weeks.

If you should find unusual changes in your mouth, try not to panic. Early diagnosis and treatment leads to a cure in 3 out of 4 cases. If a biopsy shows that abnormal cells are present, these will be removed by surgery, radiotherapy or a combination of the two. New advances in tissue grafting and repair produce an excellent cosmetic result in most cases.

CANDIDA INFECTION OF THE OESOPHAGUS

While Candida can be grown from the oesophagus of 1 in 10 healthy people, it is usually present as a normal non-harmful organism (commensal) without causing symptoms. Despite this, the oesophagus is one of the most common sites of infection in the intestinal tract. Symptoms usually occur because of an underlying problem with the immune system or with the oesophagus itself. Candida seems to prefer infecting the lower two thirds of the oesophagus – nearer the stomach – probably because this area is most likely to be damaged by acid reflux from the stomach into the gullet, which causes inflammation and heartburn. Although many people with Candidal overgrowth in the oesophagus also have oral thrush, around 1 in 3 haven't.

Candida infection of the oesophagus (gullet) is more likely if you suffer from heartburn (gastro-oesophageal reflux disease) or any condition that interferes with normal swallowing, such as:

- blockage of the oesophagus (through peptic ulceration, operative scarring, enlarged glands in the chest, thyroid goitre, tissue webs or a tumour)
- achalasia – a condition in which the oesophagus does not produce the normal muscular waves of activity during swallowing; the bottom half of the oesophagus is constricted while the upper half dilates and contains stale food
- conditions in which the soft tissues of the oesophagus become hardened (for example systemic sclerosis)
- nerve or muscle disorders in which swallowing is affected (for example myasthenia gravis, bulbar palsy, motor neurone disease)
- pouching of the oesophagus (for example diverticuli).

Sometimes, severe Candida infection of the oesophagus is caused by reduced immunity linked with a malignancy (for example leukaemia), drug treatment (such as chemotherapy, oral steroids, drugs used after transplant surgery) or AIDS. These conditions affect the way that immune cells (especially neutrophils) limit Candida infection to keep outbreaks within a limited area.

Symptoms

Candida overgrowth of the oesophagus may cause:

- difficulty swallowing
- pain on swallowing
- pain behind the breastbone (retrosternal pain)
- nausea
- vomiting
- bringing up blood (haematemesis)
- sometimes fever

In a few cases, however, it may cause no symptoms at all.

If left untreated, the raw areas may heal on their own, but this can lead to scarring and narrowing of the oesophagus, with recurrent difficulty swallowing. If you notice any symptoms that you think may be due to infection, ulceration or narrowing of the gullet, it is important to tell your doctor without delay. All symptoms should be taken seriously as, apart from anything else, other conditions such as peptic ulceration or an early cancer of the throat need to be ruled out.

Investigations

If you develop problems with swallowing, or if Candida infection is suspected, two main tests are used to investigate symptoms: a barium swallow and endoscopy.

Barium Swallow
This involves drinking a barium solution made with a flavoured liquid, or eating a biscuit or piece of bread soaked in barium. The barium drink lines the gullet so that it shows up on x-ray, while swallowing the bread/biscuit allows the swallowing pattern to be followed on a screen. By examining a series of x-rays,

a radiologist can see how well-coordinated your muscles are during swallowing, whether there is any spasm, and whether there are any obvious areas of ulceration, narrowing, dilation or abnormal blockage. While x-ray appearances may suggest a Candida infection, they cannot confirm it. Some typical appearances on x-ray include plaques separated by ulcers (which look rather like cobblestones) and severe infection of the wall of the oesophagus (giving it a shaggy, irregular outline).

Endoscopy

This involves being lightly sedated with an injection (for example with diazepam tranquillizer). Your oesophagus can then be examined with a narrow, flexible snake-like instrument (endoscope) containing a light, a camera and a tiny biopsy device. The doctor can directly view the walls of your gullet and identify any abnormal areas such as ulcers, strictures or Candida plaques. If a Candida fungal infection is found, it can be graded according to its severity:

Grade 1: scattered raised white plaques up to 2 mm in
        diameter
Grade 2: numerous plaques larger than 2 mm in diameter
Grade 3: plaques that merge together to form long white
        patches or nodules with some ulceration
Grade 4: as Grade 3, but with swelling and narrowing of the
        oesophagus and bleeding when the walls of the
        oesophagus are touched.

During endoscopy the doctor will take small biopsies for examination under the microscope. Infected areas of the oesophagus can also be brushed to provide swabs for examination and culture. This gives direct evidence of invasion of tissues by a yeast infection. Brushings seem to be more accurate than biopsies – in one study, 100 per cent of brushings taken from the oesophagus were positive for Candida, compared with only 16 per cent of biopsies performed on the same patients.

Treatment

Treatment of oesophageal Candida is usually with drugs taken by mouth. Some of these are absorbed from the gut and enter the circulation to attack the infection from the inside.

- Fluconazole (capsules or suspension): once a day for 14–30 days
- Itraconazole (capsules): once a day for 15 days (twice a day for patients with an underlying disease affecting their immunity)
- Ketoconazole: may be used where other drugs have failed; once a day for at least 1 week after symptoms have gone. Absorption of oral Ketoconazole depends on stomach acidity – treatment may fail if taken with antacids or ulcer-healing drugs.
- Amphotericin (not absorbed from the gut) is given by mouth (4 times daily) – for severe infections it may be given intravenously.

Prevention

Candida infection of the oesophagus can be minimized by avoiding heartburn and preventing acid damage to tissues in the lower oesophagus. One of the most common causes of heartburn is acid reflux, in which stomach contents reflux back up into the oesophagus. This damages and inflames the tissues lining your lower oesophagus and makes Candida infection and overgrowth more likely.

Normally, acid is stopped from coming up into the gullet by a muscle sphincter between the oesophagus and upper stomach, and by downward contractions of muscles (peristalsis) in the wall of the oesophagus. This protective mechanism may fail due to poor muscle co-ordination, weakness of the stomach sphincter, the presence of a hiatus hernia, or increased pressure on the stomach (caused, for example, by excess weight or eating too much).

Acid reflux causes hot, burning sensations in the chest that may rise up into the throat. It usually comes on within 30 minutes of eating and may be triggered by eating too much, taking exercise, bending or lying down. Meals containing fat, pastry, chocolate, acidic fruit juices, coffee or alcohol are the most common culprits. There are several self-help measures that will help to control symptoms, of which the most important are the first two in this list:

- Lose any excess weight.
- Avoid smoking cigarettes.
- Eat little and often throughout the day, rather than having 3 large meals.
- Drink fluids little and often, rather than large quantities at a time.
- Avoid hot, acid, spicy, fatty foods.
- Avoid tea, coffee and acidic fruit juices.
- Cut right back on alcohol intake – preferably avoid it altogether.
- Avoid aspirin and related drugs (for example ibuprofen).
- Avoid stooping, bending or lying down after eating.
- Avoid late-night eating.
- Elevate the head of your bed by about 15–20 cm.
- Wear loose clothing, especially around the waist.

If you suffer from recurrent indigestion or heartburn it is important to tell your doctor. A recent Gallup poll of over 1,000 people found that 48 per cent had suffered heartburn but only a quarter had sought help from their doctor or pharmacist. Seventy-five per cent of people put up with the problem or took simple remedies such as drinking milk, taking sodium bicarbonate solution or buying simple antacids over the counter. It is now known that taking antacids long term does not protect against the damage caused by acid on delicate tissues – and may also increase your risk of Candida infection. After 10–20 years, recurrent heartburn can result in scarring of the lower oesophagus with resultant difficulty in swallowing.

If symptoms of heartburn last longer than a week or two, or keep coming back, consult your doctor and tell him or her what remedies you have already tried. Your symptoms may need investigation. Research suggests that 1 in 10 people taking regular antacids – especially those over the age of 40 – could have a more serious underlying problem – including a cancer – which if picked up at an early stage is much more likely to be treated successfully.

CANDIDA INFECTION OF THE STOMACH

After the oesophagus, the stomach is the most common site of active Candida infection in the intestinal tract. Growth of Candida yeasts stop once acidity falls to a pH of 4.5, so at normal levels of acidity infection of the stomach is unusual. Candida only usually overgrows when stomach acidity drops significantly (for example when antacids are used in the treatment of peptic ulcers), when the tissues are damaged (from peptic ulcers or a tumour) or in someone with a serious illness affecting immunity (such as leukaemia, AIDS).

■ Candida can be grown from 1 in 3 biopsies taken from stomach peptic ulcers.
■ Candida can be grown from the stomach of 1 in 4 people suffering from stomach cancer.

Some doctors believe that Candida infection of peptic ulcers is so common that it should be suspected in anyone whose stomach ulcer doesn't heal with usual treatment – especially in the elderly. In one study, 5 out of 7 elderly patients with stomach ulcers did not improve with standard antacid drugs. Once they were started on an anti-fungal tablet their ulcers healed within a month.

Production of stomach acid often decreases with increasing age. This is also linked with an increased risk of Candida overgrowth in the stomach. Apart from the fact that acidity is lower, these conditions encourage production of a thicker, stickier mucus in the stomach which coats yeast cells and protects them from what little acid is present.

Symptoms

There are no typical symptoms due to active Candida infection of the stomach. Many people have no symptoms at all, while a few develop non-specific problems that can occur with any stomach disease. These symptoms include:

- loss of appetite
- weight loss
- feelings of fullness after eating very little
- burning indigestion (gastritis), triggered especially by certain foods
- nausea
- vomiting
- bringing up blood (haematemesis)
- abdominal pain
- sometimes fever.

If you develop any of these symptoms, you should tell your doctor as soon as possible.

Investigation

Stomach problems are sometimes investigated with a barium meal. You are given a barium solution to drink and then asked to lie on a table in various positions so that the solution lines your stomach. By examining a series of x-rays, a radiologist can look for areas of ulceration, growths in the stomach wall, or evidence of Candida infection such as small single or multiple ulcers, the presence of fungus balls or small cobblestone-like nodules.

If a stomach problem is suspected you are more likely to have an endoscopy these days. This is similar to the procedure described on page 81, except that the doctor will concentrate on examining your stomach and the first part of your small intestine (the upper duodenum). Biopsies will be taken from any suspicious-looking areas for examination under the microscope.

Treatment

Candida infection of the stomach can be treated with:

- Nystatin (tablets or suspension): 4–6 times daily for as long as necessary
- Fluconazole (capsules or suspension): once a day for 14–30 days
- Itraconazole (capsules): once a day for 15 days (twice a day for patients with an underlying disease affecting their immunity)
- Ketoconazole: may be used where other drugs have failed; once a day for at least 1 week after symptoms have gone. Absorption of oral Ketoconazole depends on stomach acidity – treatment may fail if taken with antacids or ulcer-healing drugs.
- Miconazole (tablets): 4 times a day for 10 days or up to 2 days after symptoms have cleared
- Amphotericin (not absorbed from the gut) is given by mouth (4 times daily) – for severe infections it may be given intravenously.

Prevention

Candida infection of the stomach can be minimized by avoiding inflammation of the stomach (gastritis or indigestion) and damage to stomach tissues.

Indigestion is a common term covering a variety of symptoms linked with eating. These include feelings of distension from swallowing air, flatulence from excessive wind in the intestines, nausea, abdominal pain and sensations of burning. Doctors refer to indigestion as dyspepsia, meaning a discomfort/burning felt centrally in the upper abdomen.

The stomach is normally protected from digesting itself by a lining of mucus that is resistant to acid attack. If this mucus lining is breached, however, acid can get through to the stomach wall and start digesting it, leading to inflammation and pain (gastritis).

Gastritis produces symptoms similar to those of a stomach ulcer, with burning or gnawing pain in the upper abdomen, nausea and vomiting. If gastritis is severe, you may even vomit and bring up blood-stained fluids (haematemesis). As the blood has usually been partly digested, it is clotted and dark, resembling dark brown tea leaves or ground coffee.

Acute gastritis can be triggered by drugs that irritate the stomach lining. These include tobacco, alcohol, and aspirin, ibuprofen and other anti-inflammatory drugs used to treat musculoskeletal problems such as arthritis or sports injuries.

Helicobacter pylori

The main cause of gastritis is now known to be infection of the stomach with a bacterium called *Helicobacter pylori*. In the UK, at least 20 per cent of 30-year-old adults and 50 per cent of those over 50 are infected. In some parts of the world up to 90 per cent of 20-year-olds are infected.

Helicobacter pylori is a mobile bacterium that can move around thanks to small whip-like propellers (flagellae). The bacteria burrows into the mucus lining of the stomach to avoid stomach acids, leaving a small breach in the wall through which acids can reach the stomach wall. *Helicobacter* then makes a special enzyme, urease, which it uses to coat itself with a small bubble of alkaline ammonia gas. This keeps the bacteria safe from acid attack and, at the same time, irritates your stomach wall leading to more inflammation. This also lets Candida yeast cells penetrate through to the gut wall so they are protected from acid attack and can start to invade your tissues if your immunity is low.

Helicobacter pylori can be diagnosed through:

- blood tests to look for antibodies to the bacteria
- breath tests – swallowing radioactive urea and breathing into a sealed bag after half an hour. If *Helicobacter* is present, its enzyme, urease, will convert urea to ammonia and radioactive ammonia will be detected in the bag.
- picking up signs of infection from saliva
- testing stomach biopsies taken during endoscopy for signs of infection.

Once diagnosed, *Helicobacter* can be eradicated by a mixture of two antibiotics plus bismuth (triple therapy) or one antibiotic plus a drug that stops the stomach from making acid (double therapy). Unfortunately, treatment (especially triple therapy) is unpleasant and can cause side-effects of sore mouth, unpleasant metallic after-taste, nausea, diarrhoea, abdominal pain and blackening of the stools and tongue. One in five patients drops out of treatment with triple therapy, although double therapy is better tolerated.

Some research from New Zealand suggests that honey made from the flower of the Manuka, or New Zealand Tea Tree, contains a unique antibiotic that can also eradicate *Helicobacter*. Taking 4 teaspoons of Manuka honey 4 times a day on an empty stomach for 8 weeks can wipe out the infection. Manuka honey is available in larger healthfood shops. If following an anti-Candida regime, however, you may wish to avoid taking honey. *NB:* If you suffer from diabetes, you should consult your doctor before using a honey treatment.

Peptic Ulcers

If erosion of the mucus lining is extensive, acid attack will lead to a raw area on the stomach wall known as a gastric ulcer. 1 in 30 adults suffers from stomach ulcers at some time in life, with men being twice as likely to develop the condition as women. It tends to come on in the age range 30–50, some 10–20 years later than duodenal ulceration. In the UK, up to a million people suffer from stomach ulcers each year, of which 9 out of 10 are a recurrence of a previous problem. Half of all patients with a stomach ulcer will have a recurrence within 2 years.

Infection with the stomach bacteria *Helicobacter pylori* is linked with 85 per cent of stomach ulcers and virtually all peptic ulcers in the duodenum (upper part of the small intestine). In addition, 1 in 3 peptic ulcers contains signs of Candida infection.

A peptic ulcer in the stomach (gastric ulcer) can produce symptoms of:

- gnawing, burning pain in the upper abdomen beneath the ribs
- pain that is usually relieved by antacids
- pain that is usually relieved by vomiting
- pain that is usually made worse by eating.

To reduce the risk of a stomach ulcer:

- Stop smoking.
- Avoid drinking alcohol, which can cause a chemical inflammation of the stomach wall (alcoholic gastritis).
- Cut right back on intakes of tea and coffee.
- Avoid aspirin and related drugs such as ibuprofen.
- Eat several small meals per day rather than 3 larger ones.
- Try to avoid stress and take regular rest and relaxation.
- Follow a relatively bland diet, avoiding foods that are excessively acidic, hot or spicy.

CANDIDA INFECTIONS OF THE SMALL INTESTINES

Normally, the contents of the jejunum (first 40 per cent of the small bowel below the duodenum) are virtually sterile. This is due to the digestive enzymes present, and the fact that the semi-solid porridge-like contents of the gut (chyme) pass through relatively quickly to flush any surviving bacteria and yeast cells through. Despite this, Candida have been isolated from the duodenal secretions of 1 in 25 healthy volunteers sampled using a naso-gastric tube, and from the jejunum of 1 in 2 apparently normal and healthy adults. As samples are taken lower and lower throughout the small intestines, the likelihood of finding Candida species increases. This implies that yeast cells can survive exposure to the strong alkaline chemicals and enzymes which join the duodenum from the bile and pancreas. The fact that Candida can survive in concentrated bile is no longer in doubt, since yeasts can be grown from up to 2 per cent of gallbladders removed at operation (cholecystectomy).

Yeasts and bacteria can survive passage through the stomach to reach the small intestines (duodenum, jejunum, ileum) if:

- your stomach empties more quickly than usual, for example if you are suffering from gastroenteritis (when food seems to go straight through you)
- a large enough quantity of yeast cells are ingested

- the yeast cells are coated and protected, for example by extra-sticky mucus
- you have a peptic ulcer that acts as a source of continual infection
- you are taking antacid preparations which reduce stomach acidity
- stomach acidity falls off (as happens with increasing age)
- you have a medical condition in which production of stomach acids is lowered (for example achlorhydria).

Candida albicans is the species most frequently grown from the small intestines, followed by *C. tropicalis*, *C. parapsilosis*, *C. stellatoidea* and *C. guillermondii* plus other closely related yeasts such as *Torulopsis glabrata*.

Symptoms

In most cases, Candida in the gut is harmless and causes no problems. If it overgrows and invades the wall of the small intestines, however, it can produce symptoms such as:

- sensitivity to certain foods
- flatulence
- bloating
- nausea
- vomiting bile-stained fluids
- abdominal pain
- diarrhoea – which is usually watery, explosive, without blood or mucus, and comes and goes over several weeks
- ulceration of the intestinal wall leading to bleeding (blood lost from this part of the bowel will usually be dark red/brown/black by the time it reaches the anus).

Most people with Candida overgrowth of the small intestines have taken broad-spectrum antibiotics or suffer from malnutrition or a serious illness that lowers their natural immunity – especially in the elderly. This is not always the case, however, and a number of apparently well people have been found to have symptoms linked with Candida overgrowth in the small intestines.

One study reported 6 cases of small bowel Candidiasis in adults, 5 of whom had no obvious underlying illness or immune problem – and only 2 of whom had recently taken antibiotics. The main symptom was diarrhoea that lasted from 4 days to 3 months. As soon as a course of anti-fungal treatment (nystatin) was started, symptoms disappeared within 3–4 days.

In another study, 50 adults with recurrent diarrhoea and a variety of gastro-intestinal symptoms were found to have a heavy growth of *Candida albicans* in their stool which was thought to be the cause of their problem.

Babies can also suffer from diarrhoea as a result of Candida infection of the small intestines. When 96 newborn babies with oral thrush were investigated, all were found to have Candida in their faeces as well. Of these, 33 babies then developed diarrhoea and, when investigated, were found to have strands of actively growing yeast colonies (hyphae and mycelium) in their bowel motions. All 33 got better with anti-fungal treatment. Six other babies developed diarrhoea but had only simple yeast cells in their stools – there were no signs of activation or overgrowth – and these did not respond to anti-fungal drugs. It is thought that diarrhoea in these 6 babies may have been linked with an allergic reaction to the yeast cells rather than to an infection itself.

Another study involving 24 babies with diarrhoea and positive stool cultures for Candida also reported that all got better within 1–8 days of starting anti-Candida treatment (nystatin).

Candida and Food Sensitivity

While overgrowth of Candida in the small intestines produces obvious inflammation which can be diagnosed and treated, the presence of non-invasive (that is, harmless) Candida in the gut is now also thought to be linked with an allergic hypersensitivity reaction. Some researchers believe this can trigger symptoms of Irritable Bowel Syndrome (IBS) – especially diarrhoea – in certain people. This may occur after taking antibiotics. Where recurrent diarrhoea is linked with hypersensitivity to yeast cells on skin testing, and where Candida are cultured from bowel motions, bowel symptoms have been shown to get worse when sufferers were given Candida extracts to eat.

Treatment to wipe out bowel Candida infection, plus a yeast-free diet (*see page 159*), have been found to help.

In many cases, however, anti-Candida treatment has not improved symptoms. Rather than dismissing Candida as a cause, researchers should instead look for another explanation in which Candida may play a role. It may be that an overgrowth of Candida has damaged the bowel wall enough to make it leaky, so that other chemicals – including partially digested food particles – which do not usually reach the bloodstream are absorbed. This may set up an immune response known as immuno-antagonism (*see page 108*). Candida overgrowth has therefore acted as a trigger for the problem even if it has not caused it directly. Once the damage is done and the bowel and immune system are sensitized to these food particles, treatment to eradicate the yeast overgrowth could not be expected to help. A diet eliminating the foods to which you are sensitive may help to solve the problem, however.

Investigation

Candida infection of the small bowel may be investigated with abdominal x-rays to look for signs of thickened and dilated loops of bowel. Endoscopic examination and small bowel biopsy will show yeast infiltration of tissues.

In severe cases, endoscopy of the duodenum and upper jejunum may reveal multiple small white patches (plaques) and ulceration in the bowel wall. This leads to swelling of the bowel lining and dilation of loops of bowel.

Occasionally, it may be necessary to take a biopsy of the lower part of the jejunum. This is achieved using a small, cylindrical device (called a Crosby capsule) that is attached to 2 metres of polyethylene tubing. The tubing is filled with saline and the capsule swallowed so that the tubing trails from the mouth as the capsule progresses through the bowel. Its position is monitored by x-ray, or positioned using an endoscopic viewing instrument. When the capsule is in the lower part of the small jejunum, a syringe is attached to the end of the tubing and suction produces a slight vacuum. This gently pulls the bowel lining up against a small hole in the capsule. A spring-loaded knife-blade within the capsule is then activated to snip off a tiny piece of the bowel lining. The capsule is then gently pulled back up through the gut to retrieve the biopsy. This test has been widely used for almost 40 years and seems to be safe. It has a few drawbacks, however:

■ It is relatively time-consuming.
■ The capsule, once withdrawn, is frequently found to be empty.
■ the capsule can become detached from its tubing during withdrawal so that the stools have to be collected and sieved for several days afterwards to retrieve the cylinder.

Treatment

Nystatin, Fluconazole, Ketoconazole, Miconazole, Amphotericin: *see page 86* for dosages.

Duodenal Ulcers

Inflammation of the duodenum (duodenitis) and duodenal ulceration increase the risk of Candida infection in the small intestines. Duodenal ulcers affect around 15 per cent of adults at some time in their life. It is most common among those aged 20–40 years. Some 60 per cent of sufferers with a duodenal ulcer will have a recurrence within 1 year.

The symptoms of duodenal ulceration include:
■ gnawing, burning pain in the upper abdomen
■ burning pain that tends to come on when hungry
■ burning pain that tends to come on at night
■ pain that is relieved by antacids
■ pain that is relieved by eating, as this triggers the release of alkaline duodenal secretions which help to neutralize excess acid in this part of the gut
■ flatulence.

Like gastric ulceration, duodenal ulcers are also linked with the bacteria *Helicobacter pylori*. Measures to help prevent duodenal ulcers are similar to those for stomach ulcers (*see page 89*).

CANDIDA INFECTIONS OF THE LARGE INTESTINES

The large intestines are made up of the colon, the rectum and the anal canal. The colon consists of 5 parts: the caecum plus appendix (counts as one), and the ascending, transverse, descending and sigmoid colon. The lining of the large bowel (mucosa) is different from that found in the small intestines – it does not contain absorption villi, only colonic glands that secrete lubricating mucus. The three muscle layers of the gut are also arranged differently in the large bowel compared with those of the stomach and small intestines. The outer layer of muscle fibres are collected together into three longitudinal bands (*taenia coli*). Because these bands are shorter than the rest of the colon, they act rather like drawstrings to pull the colonic wall into out-pouchings known as haustra. These pouches provide an ideal hiding place for bacteria and yeast cells. Mucus production is mainly stimulated by the mechanical contact of faeces with the colon wall.

Once food reaches the large bowel, most nutrients have already been absorbed. The large intestines are mainly concerned with taking up excess fluid, salts and minerals from the bowel contents. After passing through the large bowel, semi-liquid bowel contents are transformed into solidified waste matter as 90 per cent of their fluid content is absorbed – of around 2 litres of bowel contents received into the colon each day, only 200–250 ml of semi-solid waste remains for voiding.

While a few bacteria are normally found in the small intestines, it is not until the colon that masses of bacteria are seen. These bowel bacteria are usually beneficial, in that they:

- ferment and help to break down undigested fibre
- bulk up the stools to make defecation easier – over half the weight of your stools consists of bacteria
- compete for nutrients with potentially harmful bacteria and yeasts (such as Candida), which helps to stop them overgrowing
- make acids and natural antibiotics/anti-fungal substances which inhibit the growth of other organisms

- make and secrete vitamin K, B group vitamins, biotin and folic acid, which can be absorbed and used in the body
- absorb some cholesterol and fatty acids from the gut, preventing their reabsorption – when some antibiotics are given, blood cholesterol levels (especially of the more harmful LDL-cholesterol) can go up.

Candida can be grown from rectal swabs in 30 per cent of healthy people who have no symptoms of ill-health – the yeast cells are present as harmless commensals. If conditions in the large bowel change to favour Candida overgrowth (for example if normal bowel bacteria are killed by a prolonged course of antibiotics), symptoms such as bloating, loose stools and flatulence may develop. Candida can be grown from the stools of as many as 8 out of 10 people with these problems.

Symptoms

Symptoms of Candida infection of the large intestines include:

- sensitivity to certain foods
- flatulence
- bloating
- watery diarrhoea, usually without blood or excess mucus
- constipation
- uncomfortable spasm and straining when trying to pass a stool (tenesmus)
- problems similar to those of Irritable Bowel Syndrome.

Some researchers feel that diarrhoea can also be triggered in some people without an overgrowth of Candida as a result of an allergic reaction to Candida products absorbed from the bowel (*see page 91*).

Candida and Irritable Bowel Syndrome

Irritable Bowel Syndrome (IBS) is the most common condition to affect the gut. It is a problem of bowel function rather than structure, and as a result there is nothing abnormal to find during investigations and no obvious clues to help with the diagnosis. IBS is therefore referred to as a functional problem rather than an organic one. It seems to be linked with abnormal or exaggerated bowel movements and muscular spasm. To diagnose IBS, there must be *at least 3 months, continuous or recurrent symptoms of abdominal pain or discomfort which is:*

■ relieved by defecation
■ and/or associated with a change in frequency of passing stool
■ and/or associated with a change in the consistency of stool

plus two or more of the following, on at least a quarter of occasions or days:

■ altered stool frequency
■ altered stool form (lumpy/hard or loose/watery)
■ altered stool passage (straining, urgency, or feeling of incomplete evacuation)
■ passage of mucus
■ bloating or feeling of abdominal distension.

Altered stool frequency is usually taken to mean more than 3 bowel movements per day, or less than 3 bowel movements per week. Different people, however, have their own individual sense of what is normal for them, and it is this which changes in bowel habit are measured against.

Irritable Bowel Syndrome is increasingly common. At least a third of the population is affected at some time during life, even if only mildly. Overall, 15 per cent of people are affected badly enough to consult their doctor.

While overgrowth of Candida in the gut produces ulceration and inflammation which can be diagnosed and treated, the presence of non-invasive (that is, harmless) Candida in the bowel is now also thought to trigger IBS symptoms – especially diarrhoea – in certain people. This is believed to be linked with an allergic hypersensitivity reaction which may occur after a bout of gastroenteritis or taking antibiotics. Both disrupt the normal balance of bacteria found in the bowel, affect the normal process of fermentation in the colon, and change the amount and composition of bowel gases produced.

Many people with IBS develop symptoms for the first time after an attack of gastroenteritis (bowel infection). During 1994, 38 victims of an outbreak of Salmonella food poisoning were studied by researchers; over the next year, almost a third (12 out of 38–32 per cent) went on to develop recurrent bowel symptoms consistent with IBS. In most cases, they developed intermittent diarrhoea. Those with the worst symptoms of gastroenteritis (diarrhoea lasting longer than 7 days plus vomiting leading to weight loss) were more likely to develop IBS than those with milder symptoms. They were also the ones who took longer to recover their appetite, weight and energy levels.

Another study looked at 75 patients who developed gastroenteritis (from various organisms) that was bad enough for them to be admitted to hospital. Of these, 22 (29 per cent) had symptoms 3 months later that were consistent with IBS. Nine out of 10 of these were still suffering after 6 months, and three-quarters still had IBS problems 1 year later. As in the first study, those with the worst symptoms (longer-lasting diarrhoea, with abdominal pain and mucus in the stools) were more likely to develop IBS.

Researchers are unclear why bacterial bowel infections are linked with IBS, but a sensitivity to Candida products, or to a yeast overgrowth which somehow interferes with normal bowel function, have been suggested as possibilities.

While taking a course of antibiotics, it is worth eating live (unpasteurized) BIO yoghurt containing organisms such as *Lactobacillus acidophilus*, or a drink (sold as Yakult) containing *Lactobacillus casei* Shirota. There is evidence that these bacteria can survive the journey through the stomach and small intestines to reach the bowel and recolonize the large intestines with friendly bacteria. This can help to damp down Candida overgrowth. Many IBS sufferers claim that eating BIO yoghurt every day keeps their symptoms under control – whether they have recently taken antibiotics or not.

Altogether, bowel micro-organisms – including yeasts – make up around 30 per cent of normal stool bulk:

Stools contain:

water   75 per cent
solids   25 per cent

Of which:

- around 30 per cent = bacteria and some yeasts
- around 15 per cent = inorganic material (for example calcium and phosphates)
- around 5 per cent = fats
- a varying amount is undigested plant fibre (roughage) depending on diet
- a small amount of desquamated (shed) bowel lining cells, mucus and digestive enzymes.

Investigation

Investigation of large bowel symptoms may involve:

- an abdominal examination
- a digital (finger) rectal examination
- stool cultures to look for bacteria or Candida – although if yeast cells are found they may not be reported if they are in their simple cell form (no hyphae) and are assumed to be a normal part of the bowel flora
- testing for hidden blood (faecal occult blood) which may be a sign of inflammation or possibly a tumour
- ultrasound to look for abnormal masses
- proctoscopy – insertion of a speculum to examine the inner walls of the rectum to look for inflammation or ulceration
- sygmoidoscopy – insertion of a tube with a light on the end to examine the inner lining of the lower (sigmoid) colon and to biopsy any lesions seen
- colonoscopy – insertion of a longer, flexible instrument similar to a sigmoidoscope, to inspect further up the colon. You will be given a powerful laxative (or oral bowel cleansing solution) to take beforehand which acts within 10–14 hours. This helps to empty the bowel and provide a better view. You will probably be sedated during the procedure.
- a barium enema – coating the bowel lining with a substance that shows up on x-ray, such as barium sulphate. Before

having a barium enema you will be asked not to eat anything the night before, and to drink plenty of fluids instead. You will also be given a powerful laxative to empty your bowel so that faeces don't get in the way of the test.
- a test for deficiency of the enzyme, lactase – which can also cause symptoms such as bowel distension, pain, flatulence and diarrhoea.

Where recurrent diarrhoea is linked with hypersensitivity to yeast cells on skin testing (not often performed on the NHS) and where Candida are cultured from bowel motions, bowel symptoms have been shown to get worse on being given Candida extracts to eat. Treatment to wipe out bowel Candida infection, plus a yeast-free diet (*see page 159*) may help.

Treatment

Nystatin, Fluconazole, Ketoconazole, Miconazole, Amphotericin: *see page 86* for dosages.

Prevention

Try to eat more fibre – every gram of dietary fibre increases stool weight by around 5 g. This is because fibre provides fermentable food for bacteria, allowing them to grow and divide – to compete with Candida cells. Fibre is also thought to bind Candida toxins in the gut, helping to move yeast cells downwards; this may relieve symptoms.

Drink plenty of fluids to bulk up dietary fibre.

Eat natural BIO yoghurt containing *Lactobacillus acidophilus*, or a drink containing *Lactobacillus casei* Shirota.

Stop smoking, and try to avoid passive smoking, too. Receptors in the gut react with nicotine and affect bowel function, which may make symptoms worse.

Increase the amount of exercise you take. This improves bowel function and can help to relieve symptoms of bloating and distension.

Try to avoid unnecessary stress – the intestines contain receptors which interact with stress hormones and can make symptoms worse.

Try following an anti-Candida diet (*see Chapter 10*) to see if this helps.

ANAL ITCHING

Everyone suffers from anal itching at some time in life – in the UK, around half a million people receive treatment for the condition each year. For some reason, it seems to attack men more than women. It is usually worse at night and when increased sweating occurs – as a result of central heating being set at too high a temperature, warm weather, taking part in vigorous sport, or sitting for long periods of time. There are many different causes:

- thrush (fungal infection)
- poor hygiene after opening the bowels
- wearing tight, nylon underwear
- threadworms
- an allergy to cloth dyes or washing powders
- eating spicy foods
- drinking excessive amounts of caffeine
- haemorrhoids (piles)
- anal fissures
- anal skin tags
- genital warts
- infestations such as scabies or pubic lice
- skin diseases such as eczema or psoriasis
- other medical problems such as diabetes, anaemia or vitamin deficiency.

In half of all cases, no obvious cause is found.

Even if an itchy bottom isn't originally due to a Candida infection, it will soon lead to anal thrush if constant scratching damages the surrounding skin. Candida is present in the faeces of up to 80 per cent of the population and will rapidly overgrow when skin is broken and conditions are warm and moist.

Symptoms

- intense itching
- soreness, especially on wiping the bottom
- moist discharge
- weeping sores
- discomfort on opening the bowels
- difficulty opening the bowels
- worsening of symptoms due to piles.

Investigation

In most cases, no investigations are necessary. A swab may be sent for analysis if a diagnosis of thrush is not obvious – this will also help to pick up a bacterial infection and threadworm eggs.

Treatment

Anal itching caused by Candida is treated with anti-fungal creams such as Clotrimazole. For non-infective itching, or itching due to haemorrhoids (piles), over-the-counter remedies such as Anusol, Germaloids, Hemocane or Preparation H can be used. In general, a cream formulation is less messy and uncomfortable than an ointment, although an ointment is more soothing if you are sore or have intense itching.

If symptoms persist for more than a few days, do consult your doctor. Stronger agents are available on prescription – including a new spray treatment (Perinal) containing a local anaesthetic and an anti-inflammatory agent.

Prevention

- Bathe or shower every day using unperfumed soap.
- Use wet wipes and soft toilet roll – not rough, medicated paper.
- Wipe your bottom correctly (from front to back).
- Wash the area with unperfumed soap after every bowel movement – using water alone will not remove greasy residues.

- Dry the anus thoroughly by patting it gently with a soft towel (a rough one will only make matters worse) – or use a hair-dryer set on gentle heat.
- Wear loose cotton underwear, changing it at least once per day.
- Avoid using talcum powder – although an anti-fungal powder spray can be helpful.
- Eat a mild, non-spicy diet and go easy on caffeine.
- If you keep scratching at night, try wearing cotton underwear and even cotton gloves.
- Take steps to reduce Candida colonization of your bowel (*see page 86*).

Threadworms

A threadworm infestation involves a small, parasitic worm called *Enterobius vermicularis*. Threadworms are also known as pinworms, as the mature female has a blunt head and a long, thin, pointed tail. Threadworms commonly infect the gut; as many as one in five children may carry them at any one time. The female threadworm is around 1 cm long and white. She comes out of the anus, mainly at night, to lay her eggs; she may deposit as many as 10,000 in one go. This causes a strong tickling sensation which makes you scratch, often in your sleep. Eggs are then deposited on the fingers and frequently transferred back to the mouth to set up a cycle of (faeco-oral) infection. Eggs can also be passed on to toys, blankets, etc., where they may survive for up to 3 weeks, increasing the chance of infecting others. Diagnosis is simple as the worms can usually be seen around the anus and on the surface of bowel motions.

Apart from causing itching, threadworms do not seem to cause any harm. If you can stop scratching at night, the infection will disappear spontaneously within a few weeks. Ointments can stop anal itching, or a drug treatment, piperazine, can be bought from pharmacies. The dose needs to be repeated after 2 weeks. The whole family may need to be treated.

BREAKING THE RE-INFESTATION CYCLE

- Wear pyjamas to minimize direct scratching of the anus.
- Have a bath/shower every morning to remove eggs laid overnight.
- Change sheets and nightwear frequently (nightly if possible).
- Wash sheets and nightwear at high temperatures, then press with a hot iron to kill the eggs.
- Keep fingernails short.
- Wash hands thoroughly and scrub with a nailbrush after visiting the bathroom and before each meal.
- Eating garlic, carrots and pumpkin seeds are all said to help clear the infection.
- Herbalists may prescribe Wormwood, Tansy or Male Fern, which have purgatives that can help to clear the infection.

Chapter Seven

SYSTEMIC AND CHRONIC CANDIDA INFECTION

SYSTEMIC CANDIDA

The most serious type of Candida infection is systemic Candidiasis, in which yeast cells spread throughout the body to infect two or more organs such as the liver, kidneys, lungs, heart, spleen or brain. As you can imagine, this only usually occurs where there is a major breakdown in immune defences.

Candida yeasts mainly enter the body from the intestines. This is known as translocation and was first proved by a brave doctor volunteer who drank a solution containing 1 billion Candida yeast cells. He developed signs of blood infection (fever and shakes) within 3 hours. Yeast cells were found in his bloodstream and urine within 6 hours.

Further research suggests that live yeast cells can move across the bowel lining into the bloodstream and lymphatic system from all parts of the digestive system, but mainly from the jejunum in the small intestines. Blood from the intestines contains absorbed nutrients and travels straight to the liver, so this is usually the first organ to show signs of a systemic Candida infection (for example small abscesses), closely followed by the spleen, which filters cells and infections from the blood. Candida yeast cells can also cross into the circulation from the lungs, but this is thought to account for only 3 per cent of systemic Candida infections.

Usually, Candida yeast cells only enter the circulation if:

■ a very large number of organisms are present and swamp the system
■ the normal bacterial content of the gut is disrupted leading

to Candida overgrowth (for example after a prolonged course of antibiotics)
- the immune system is suppressed (for example by drugs or illness)
- the lining of the gut is damaged (for example by peptic ulceration)
- blood flow to the gut wall is reduced (for example in the case of shock).

When only a small number of yeast cells are involved, these are usually quickly mopped up by macrophage scavenger cells or neutrophil pus cells, unless the immune system is under strain. As a result, systemic Candidiasis usually only develops in people who have:

- cancer – especially one involving the blood such as leukaemia or lymphoma
- poor immunity due to drug treatment (for example for organ transplants or cancer)
- had a major operation and are on intravenous antibiotics
- AIDS.

Treatment

Options include:

- Itraconazole by mouth
- Ketoconazole by mouth
- Flucytosine by intravenous injection
- Amphotericin by intravenous injection
- Fluconazole by intravenous injection.

CHRONIC CANDIDA INFECTION

For many years *Candida albicans* was thought to be a relatively harmless organism, or one that only caused nuisance problems such as recurrent vaginal thrush. More and more people are now convinced that a large number of common symptoms are linked with a chronic (long-term) sensitivity to *Candida albicans* yeasts. This is known as the Candida hypersensitivity syndrome. These recurrent symptoms may include:

- fatigue
- tiredness all the time
- irritability
- anxiety
- depression
- insomnia
- difficulty concentrating
- headache
- joint and muscle pains
- sugar and carbohydrate cravings
- recurrent cystitis where no evidence of infection is found
- Irritable Bowel Syndrome (IBS)
- alcohol intolerance
- problems after taking antibiotics.

Despite the fact that this is a controversial area, many researchers and doctors are starting to believe that Candida hypersensitivity, or some form of food intolerance, is linked with other long-term problems such as:

- pre-menstrual syndrome
- chronic fatigue syndrome (also known as ME)
- asthma
- eczema
- arthritis
- IBS
- cellulite.

These symptoms and conditions are not due to an overgrowth of Candida or invasion of tissues with yeast cells as such, and anti-fungal treatments do not seem to help.

Some researchers have suggested that the problem is due to an oversensitivity of the immune system to Candida proteins. These are absorbed from the gut into the bloodstream and interact with antibodies and immune cells to trigger symptoms.

These antibodies may persist and attack other parts of the body to continue causing problems even when the original Candida infection is long gone. Although there is no proof of this at present it is known that, in conditions in which antibodies bind to foreign proteins to form circulating soluble complexes, symptoms such as fatigue and feeling non-specifically unwell (malaise) usually occur.

It is also possible that the normal presence of Candida yeast cells living relatively harmlessly in the gut makes the intestinal lining more leaky, so that incompletely digested food particles can enter the circulation more easily. Once this leakiness has occurred, the immune system may become sensitized to these food particles to produce a variety of symptoms. This would explain why anti-fungal drugs do not seem to improve the problem.

Food Allergy and Intolerance

Food intolerance and allergy is an interesting but controversial topic. Food intolerance is defined as a reproducible, adverse reaction to a specific food or ingredient which occurs even when the food is eaten in a disguised form. It is relatively common. In contrast, a food allergy is a relatively rare form of food intolerance in which an abnormal immune response triggers a potentially devastating chain of reactions in the body, often involving the production of histamine and a type of antibody called IgE.

There are several medically accepted types of food intolerance and allergy, including:

- severe anaphylactic reaction – with life-threatening symptoms (falling blood pressure, difficulty breathing, tissue swelling) triggered by foods such as peanuts
- hypersensitivity – with widespread, itchy rash (urticaria), eczema, asthma, vomiting, abdominal pains or diarrhoea when eating foods such as strawberries, eggs or shellfish
- food sensitivity – chemicals in chocolate, cheese or red wine, for example, can trigger migraine
- lactose intolerance – due to the inability to digest lactose

sugar in milk, causing bloating, abdominal pain and diarrhoea

■ gluten intolerance – causing bloating, abdominal pain, bulky stools, malabsorption and weight loss (coeliac disease).

The type of food reaction that has been linked with Candida is different from these, and is not really an allergy at all. It is closer to a food intolerance; some researchers have labelled it an immuno-antagonism. The area is controversial, but the theory goes that when food is eaten, it is broken down in the intestines into small building-blocks (proteins are broken down into amino acids, fats into fatty acids and carbohydrates into simple sugars) before being absorbed. In some cases, however, it is thought that certain foods, to which your immune system is sensitive, make your intestinal wall porous. It is thought that this leakiness may be linked to the presence of Candida cells. This lets incompletely digested food particles enter your bloodstream. This theory is supported by research in which proteins from egg yolk and cow's milk have been found in human breastmilk. The only logical way in which they could have got there was through the bloodstream from the gut.

Once in the circulation, food particles to which you are sensitive are quickly attacked by the immune system, coated by immune proteins and destroyed by white blood cells called neutrophils (pus cells). If you eat too many of the foods to which you are sensitive, however, it is thought that your immune system becomes swamped. You run out of complement proteins, and incompletely coated food particles are free to roam around your body. This challenge to the immune system has been linked with feelings of being tired all the time. The food particles are eventually filtered out in the kidney and destroyed, but may set up immune reactions in different parts of the body linked with the chronic illnesses mentioned above.

At present this is just a theory and there is no firm evidence to confirm it, although much research continues in the area.

Researchers have found that the people most likely to have a food sensitivity and who respond best to avoiding certain foods (for example by following an anti-Candida diet) are those who suffer from chronic diarrhoea.

Elimination Diet

The diagnosis of food intolerance and allergy can only be made with any degree of reliability when symptoms disappear during an elimination diet and reappear when the suspected food is reintroduced – even in a hidden form.

There are several degrees of an exclusion diet:

- simple exclusion, with the elimination of a single food
- multiple exclusion – elimination of several foods which have been linked with a particular health problem
- restriction diet – which consists of eating very few foods, for example nothing but a single meat (for example lamb), a single source of carbohydrate (such as rice) and a single fruit (for example pears) and drinking only spring, mineral or distilled water.

After following the elimination diet until symptoms have disappeared (commonly 10–21 days), the eliminated foods are reintroduced one by one, usually at 3-day intervals, to see which triggers a recurrence. You will need to keep a careful food and symptom diary during this time. Following an elimination diet is time-consuming, can be boring, and requires a great deal of motivation.

There are many other tests that can be arranged to test for food sensitivity.

Sublingual Testing

A few drops of a solution containing the food to which you are thought to be intolerant (and which you haven't eaten recently) are placed under your tongue and your response noted. There is a possible risk of an anaphylactic reaction if you are highly sensitive to the food (for example peanuts) and swelling of the tongue and throat may occur, although this is rare. In most cases, unfortunately, this test proves inconclusive.

Food Challenge Tests

The food to which you are thought to be sensitive is given orally and your response noted. This can be helpful in establishing whether a particular food triggers symptoms but where there is a risk of a severe allergic response (anaphylaxis). It should only be carried out under close medical supervision.

Skin Contact Tests
These are sometimes used to investigate food allergies. A diluted extract is placed on the skin, and if a reaction occurs, allergy is said to be present. No one is sure how useful these tests are, as many false results occur.

Skin Prick Tests
A substance you are thought to be allergic to is applied to the skin; the substance is then pricked into your skin with a fine, sterile needle. Measuring the size of weal produced shows how severe the reaction is – for a positive result, a visible skin reaction usually covers an area at least 1 cm square around the injection site. False results (positive and negative) are common, so results should be interpreted with caution. When performed by a specialist, the area showing the skin reaction may be biopsied, stained and examined under a microscope to look for the presence of immune cells. Skin tests in which an allergic substance is pricked into the lower levels of the skin (intradermal tests) can prove dangerous, as they may trigger a severe allergic reaction.

Hair and Nail Analysis
While this may provide useful information on vitamin and mineral deficiencies, it has no proven benefit in helping to diagnose food intolerance.

Pulse Testing
Some researchers believe that, after eating a food to which you are intolerant, your pulse rate will go up. This is not reliable, however, as many factors affect the pulse rate, including anxiety, exercise, certain drugs and smoking cigarettes.

Antibody Screening
This can detect true allergy by looking for special allergy antibodies known as IgE. The technique, known as RAST (radioallergosorbent test), measures specific IgE antibody levels in

response to the suspected allergen. Unfortunately the test is not that sensitive – false positives and negatives occur, so results must be interpreted with caution. Some patients with little specific IgE may have severe allergic symptoms, while someone with lots of specific IgE can have few symptoms.

The LEAP Test

A sample of blood is split and incubated with 50 or 100 food extracts for $1\frac{1}{2}$ hours. All the white cells in the sample are then analysed to see if they have changed in size. If the white cells (neutrophils) in a sample have changed in size by more than 9 per cent, or if they have disintegrated, it suggests you are sensitive to that food. You can also be tested for sensitivity to 20 natural and man-made chemicals and fungi, including Candida.

This testing is controversial. For more information about the LEAP programme, contact Oxford Nutritional Services on 01703 222007.

NuTron Test

This takes food intolerance testing even further. A sample of blood is split and incubated with 92 food extracts (including yeasts) for 1 hour. The neutrophils in the sample are then analysed. As well as determining whether they become larger, smaller or disintegrate, radio-frequency waves and direct current testing detects other changes inside the cells (such as the formation of vacuoles, granulation) which would be missed by simply measuring cell volume. If any changes are found, you are said to be sensitive to that food.

This testing is controversial. For more information, phone NuTron Laboratories on 01483 203555.

Food Allergen Cellular Test (FACT)

Immune cells (including neutrophils, basophils, eosinophils) are incubated with food samples and the chemicals released by the cells are analysed to determine which foods you are sensitive to.

This testing is controversial. For more information about FACT, contact the Institute of Individual Well-Being, 0171–495 7040.

Other recurrent problems linked with food intolerance include:
- migraine
- eczema and psoriasis
- rheumatoid arthritis
- depression
- tinnitus
- fluid retention and weight gain
- palpitations and breathlessness
- nasal congestion (rhinitis)
- myalgic encephalomyelitis (ME)

Chronic Mucocutaneous Candida

Some people with chronic recurrent Candida infections do suffer from an obvious Candida overgrowth which can be confirmed by finding activated yeast cells in the hyphae form. This is known as Chronic Mucocutaneous Candidiasis. It can affect any one of any age, but sufferers commonly fall into the following groups:

- infants under the age of 3 – with persistent or recurrent nappy rash and/or oral thrush with widespread skin involvement
- teenagers – possibly linked with taking long-term antibiotics for acne, which allows the growth of Candida in the intestinal tract or vagina
- young adults – possibly linked with use of inhaled steroids for asthma, with an abnormality of the thymus (a gland in the chest where immune T-cells are programmed) or with HIV
- women of reproductive age with recurrent vaginal thrush – may be linked with iron deficiency
- women of reproductive age with chronic mouth Candidiasis but no skin or nail problems – linked with iron deficiency
- older people with chronic mouth problems – linked to wearing dentures (denture stomatitis).

These chronic Candida infections involve the skin, nails and mucous membranes and may be hereditary in some families.

Infections respond to taking oral anti-fungal treatments – mouth thrush clears in 5–7 days and skin lesions improve within 2 weeks as normal, but signs of infection usually recur soon after treatment is stopped.

Research suggests that most people with chronic Candidiasis have defects in their immunity which make them more susceptible to infection of yeast cells. These defects are thought to involve the T lymphocytes, neutrophils (pus cells) or macrophages (scavenger cells), although some people have abnormalities with their B lymphocytes and antibody production.

Some sufferers have been found to have one or more poorly functioning endocrine (hormone) glands such as the thymus, adrenals, parathyroids, thyroid or ovaries.

A few people with chronic Candida infection develop patchy loss of skin pigmentation (vitiligo) or loss of hair (alopecia). This may affect a small area (alopecia areata) or be widespread (for example alopecia totalis).

One in five people with chronic recurrent Candidiasis also has recurrent problems with other types of fungal infections such as dermatophytes (*see page 27*). Others have repeated and often severe viral or bacterial chest infections.

Although sufferers develop recurrent Candida infections of the skin, nails and mucous membranes – including those in the gut – they do not seem to develop serious Candida invasion of the blood or organs (systemic Candidiasis).

Treatment

A variety of treatments has been tried to help overcome Chronic Mucocutaneous Candidiasis. These include long-term, daily use of anti-fungal mouth treatments such as lozenges, pastilles or gel for recurrent oral thrush, weekly use of pessaries for recurrent vaginal thrush and regular use of anti-fungal creams if only a small area of skin is affected. For more widespread problems, long-term treatment with anti-fungal tablets or capsules is needed, although there is a risk of side-effects (*see Chapter 8*) or the development of resistance to treatment. Symptoms will unfortunately return if treatment is stopped.

Various experimental treatments are being tried to correct the immune deficiency that causes an increased susceptibility to Candida. These include immunoglobulin, transplantation of bone marrow or thymus tissues, immune transfer factors and gene therapy.

An anti-Candida diet (*see Chapter 10*) will often help to improve symptoms by reducing the number of Candida cells present in the gut.

Chapter Eight

ANTI-CANDIDA DRUGS

Anti-Candida treatments mainly work by making fungal cell walls leaky, so yeasts swell with water, lose some of their contents, and quickly die.

Candida infections are usually treated with either a topical skin cream/gel/ointment, a pessary or concentrated cream for insertion into the vagina, or a tablet/suspension/capsule taken by mouth. In serious infections (for example systemic Candidiasis), an intravenous drug may be needed.

This chapter looks at some anti-fungal drugs, giving information on possible side-effects, those for whom the drugs may not be suitable, and which medications the drugs interact with. If you develop any side-effects that you think may be linked with your medication – even if not listed here – always tell your doctor. Do not take any drugs if you are pregnant or breastfeeding, except under medical advice.

TOPICAL PREPARATIONS

With topical preparations, the risk of side-effects is small and usually only involves mild burning – especially when applied to raw, inflamed skin or mucous membranes – and sometimes irritation. Hypersensitivity reactions such as itching, redness, swelling and an allergic-type rash may occasionally occur, but this is rare. Some creams (for example nystatin) may cause weakening or destruction of rubber contraceptive diaphragms or condoms.

ORAL DRUGS

If you need to take an oral anti-fungal agent and are already taking other medications – including those bought over the counter – always check with a pharmacist or doctor that the drugs will not interact.

Amphotericin

Amphotericin is not absorbed from the gut and, when given orally to treat intestinal yeast infections, is usually tolerated quite well. It can also be given into the veins to treat systemic Candidiasis, but does not penetrate body tissues very well and commonly causes side-effects by this route – a small test dose to check for sensitivity reactions is important. One preparation, in which amphotericin is bound to fat globules (liposomes), is much less toxic when given into the veins.

Possible side-effects of intravenous amphotericin include nausea and vomiting, diarrhoea, abdominal pain, fever, headache, muscle and joint pains, anaemia, salt imbalances, nerve problems (including hearing loss or fits), liver and kidney problems, allergic reactions, irritation at injection site.

Amphotericin should not be used during pregnancy or breastfeeding.

Fluconazole

Possible side-effects of fluconazole include gastro-intestinal symptoms (for example nausea, diarrhoea, flatulence, pain), rash and allergic reactions (rare).

Should not be taken during pregnancy or breastfeeding – nor by those with kidney problems except under medical supervision.

Oral fluconazole interacts with some drugs including anticoagulants, and with some drugs used to treat epilepsy, asthma or breathing problems, diabetes and heartburn/indigestion.

Intravenous fluconazole can be given for systemic Candidiasis.

Flucytosine

Given by intravenous injection to treat systemic Candidiasis. Tablets may also be used by certain patients.

Possible side-effects of flucytosine include gastric upsets, confusion, hallucinations, fits, headache, dizziness, sleepiness, liver or blood problems.

Should not be used in people with liver or kidney problems without monitoring blood tests. Should only be used cautiously in pregnancy or when breastfeeding.

Griseofulvin

Griseofulvin is inactive when used topically, but when taken by mouth is well absorbed from the gut and is taken up by cells containing keratin (skin, hair, nails). It must be used for several weeks or months to cure an infection, but side-effects are uncommon. Possible ones include headache, nausea, vomiting, allergic reactions, dizziness, fatigue, confusion, blood abnormalities, sensitivity to light, reduced tolerance to alcohol. Lupus erythematosus, erythema multiforme and epidermal necrolysis have rarely been reported.

Griseofulvin should not be taken by those with porphyria, liver disease or SLE, or during pregnancy.

Griseofulvin interacts with some drugs, including alcohol, anticoagulants, barbiturates and oral contraceptives.

Itraconazole

Possible side-effects with oral Itraconazole include nausea, abdominal pain, indigestion, constipation, headache, dizziness, period problems and allergic reactions. In long-term treatment, jaundice fluid retention or hair loss have been reported, albeit rarely.

Oral Itraconazole should not be used during pregnancy or breastfeeding. It is important to take proper contraceptive precautions before, during and for 1 month after taking a course of treatment. It should only be used with caution in people with liver problems.

Itraconazole can interact with some drugs, including antacids and some antihistamines.

Ketoconazole

Possible side-effects of oral ketoconazole include gastric upsets, rashes, headache, allergic reactions, altered liver function, nerve problems, low platelet count and breast enlargement plus low sperm count in males (rare). People taking ketoconazole usually have their liver function checked by blood tests at regular intervals after the first 2 weeks of treatment. Oral ketoconazole should not be used for superficial fungal infections because of the risk of liver damage during use.

Should not be taken during pregnancy or by people with liver problems.

Ketoconazole interacts with some other drugs, including antacids, some anti-epilepsy treatments and antihistamines. Absorption of oral ketoconazole depends on stomach acidity – treatment may fail if taken with antacids or ulcer-healing drugs.

Ketoconazole cream and shampoos are only available on prescription at NHS expense for people with seborrhoeic dermatitis, (for example dandruff) or pityriasis versicolor.

Miconazole

Possible side-effects of oral treatment include nausea and vomiting, itching and allergic rashes.

Oral tablets or gel should only be used under medical advice during pregnancy, and should be avoided by people with porphyria.

Miconazole interacts with some drugs, including anticoagulants, anticonvulsants, some anti-diabetes drugs, cisapride and amphotericin.

Nystatin

Nystatin is not absorbed from the gut when given by mouth. It is too toxic to be given intravenously.

Possible side-effects from oral nystatin include nausea, vomiting, diarrhoea, irritation, rash.

Oral nystatin should not be used during pregnancy or breast-feeding except under close medical supervision.

Terbinafine

Possible side-effects of oral terbinafine include stomach discomfort, loss of appetite, nausea, diarrhoea, headache, rash, joint pains, skin sensitivity, taste disturbance and jaundice (rare).

Should not be taken by people with liver or kidney problems, or during pregnancy or breastfeeding.

Terbinafine interacts with some drugs, including ulcer-healing drugs (cimetidine).

Chapter Nine

COMPLEMENTARY TREATMENTS

Many people suffering symptoms of chronic or recurrent Candida infection seek help from alternative therapists. There are many reasons for this:

- Those with symptoms of Candida infections may feel their doctor is uninterested in the problem – in contrast, alternative practitioners take a holistic approach, which minimizes some patients' sense of abandonment.
- Sufferers are often left feeling that their problems are due to an emotional cause which a holistic approach may be more successful in treating.
- Orthodox medicine may be able to improve Candida symptoms for a short while, but in many cases the problems recur – it is then only natural to seek relief from the many complementary therapies available.
- Alternative treatments are often helpful in relieving Candida symptoms without the side-effects associated with some drugs.

Before trying alternative treatments for your symptoms, make sure you have been fully investigated and the diagnosis of Candida has been confirmed by your doctor – sometimes other conditions can mimic recurrent thrush (for example anaerobic vaginosis, oral leukoplakia, Irritable Bowel Syndrome, skin diseases) and it is important that the correct diagnosis is made.

When choosing an alternative practitioner, bear in mind that standards of training and experience vary widely. Where possible:

- Select a therapist on the basis of personal recommendation from a satisfied client whom you know and whose opinion you trust.
- Check what qualifications the therapist has, and check his or her standing with the relevant umbrella organization for that therapy. This organization will be able to tell you what training their members have undertaken and their code of ethics, and can refer you to qualified practitioners in your area.
- Find out how long your course of treatment will last and how much it is likely to cost.
- Ask how much experience the practitioner has had in treating Candida, and about his or her success rate.

The following complementary therapies have helped many people with recurrent or chronic Candida but, just as with orthodox medicine, not every treatment will suit every individual.

ACUPUNCTURE

Acupuncture is based on the belief that life energy (*chi* or *qi*) flows through the body along 12 different channels called meridians. When this energy flow becomes blocked, symptoms of illness are triggered. By inserting fine needles into specific acupuncture points overlying these meridians, blockages are overcome and the flow of *qi* corrected or altered to relieve symptoms. Altogether, there are 365 acupoints in the body; your therapist will select which points to use depending on your individual symptoms. Fine, disposable needles are used, which cause little if any discomfort. You may notice a slight pricking sensation, or an odd tingling buzz as the needle is inserted a few millimetres into the skin. The needles are usually left in place for up to 20 minutes, and may be twiddled periodically. Sometimes a small cone of dried herbs is ignited and burned near the active acupoint to warm the skin. This is known as moxibustion. The best known effect of *qi* manipulation is pain relief (local anaesthesia). Research suggests that acupuncture causes the release of heroin-like chemicals (endorphins) in the body which act as natural painkillers. Acupuncture can be effective in treating the symptoms of Candida.

Acupressure is similar to acupuncture, but instead of inserting needles at selected points along the meridians, these points are stimulated using firm thumb pressure or fingertip massage. The best-known example of acupressure is Shiatsu massage.

AROMATHERAPY

The following oils have anti-fungal properties and can be diluted to massage into affected areas, or added to water to bathe lesions or help to prevent recurrences:

- Bergamot
- Cajeput
- German Chamomile (do not use during first 3 months of pregnancy)
- Eucalyptus oil
- Geranium (do not use during pregnancy)
- Lavender (not during first 3 months of pregnancy)
- Lemon
- Marjoram (not during pregnancy)
- Myrrh (not during pregnancy)
- Niaouli
- Palmarosa
- Patchouli
- Rosemary (do not use if you suffer from epilepsy or are pregnant)
- Tea Tree
- Thyme (not during pregnancy)
- Yarrow.

Always use aromatherapy oils in a diluted form (for example by adding to a carrier oil) as some neat oils can irritate tissues, especially ones that are already inflamed by a Candida infection. There are a few exceptions – small amounts of Rosemary or Lavender oils can be used neat on the skin as long as they don't irritate.

For Oral Thrush

- Rinse your mouth with a home-made mouthwash made by adding 3 drops Tea Tree and 1 drop Myrrh essential oils to a small glass of water. Stir the solution vigorously before using 3 times a day. Alternatively, use tincture of Myrrh.

For Vulvo-vaginal Thrush

- Add 5 drops each Tea Tree, Myrrh and Lavender to 30 ml carrier oil and add to your bath water. Lie in the water and soak for 20 minutes.

For Vulvo-vaginal Itching

- Add 2 drops of Tea Tree, Myrrh or Lavender to a little vitamin E cream, live Bio yoghurt or KY jelly and apply to the vulval area. Use as often as necessary to relieve symptoms.

For Itching around the Anus

- Add 5 drops each of Bergamot, Lavender and Geranium to 30 ml carrier oil. Add to your bath and soak for 20 minutes, or add a few drops to warm water and use to bathe the affected area as often as necessary.

For Balanitis

- Add 4 drops Tea Tree oil and 4 drops Lavender or Patchouli oil to a bowl of warm water and use to wash under the foreskin twice a day. Add the same oils to 30 ml carrier oil (preferably Jojoba) and apply to the end of the penis at night.

For Fungal Infections of Skin Folds

- Add 10 drops Eucalyptus and 5 drops Lavender to 30 ml carrier oil and add to bath water. Lie back and soak the affected area (groin, under the breasts) for 20 minutes. Add the same oils to a bowl of warm water and bathe the affected area twice a day.
- Use an aromatherapy dusting powder (*see below*) to keep skin folds fresh and dry after bathing.

For Fungal Infections of the Groin

- Dissolve 2 drops of Lavender, Cypress, Tea Tree or Patchouli oil in 30 ml carrier oil and apply to the area twice a day.
- Also add one or more of these oils to your bath water.

For Athlete's Foot

- Clean out debris from under and around the toenails (where infection often lurks), then bathe the cleaned foot in water to which you have added a few drops of Lavender, Myrrh, Palmarosa or Tea Tree essential oils.
- Add 1 drop of Lavender, Myrrh, Palmarosa or Tea Tree to 1 tablespoon of Calendula or Chamomile cream. Mix well and rub into the affected area.
- If the area is very moist, dissolve one or more of the above oils in surgical spirits and apply for a few days until the skin dries out.
- Use an aromatherapy dusting powder (*see below*) to keep feet fresh and dry after bathing – dust the inside of your shoes and socks with this powder, too.

For Ringworm on the Body

- Add 1 drop each of Myrrh, Lavender and Tea Tree essential oils to 1 tablespoon of Calendula or Chamomile cream and mix. Apply to skin lesions 3 times a day.
- 1 drop of neat Rosemary oil can be rubbed into small areas of skin if preferred.

For Ringworm on the Scalp

- Rub the scalp with a solution of Rosemary oil in water if scalp is dry. If lesions are moist, or scalp is greasy, add the Rosemary oil to a little surgical spirits and rub into the affected area once or twice a day.

Anti-fungal Dusting Powder

- 150 g pharmaceutical grade talc (from a chemist)
- 15 drops Tea Tree oil
- 10 drops Lavender
- 10 drops Rosemary
- 5 drops Bergamot

Mix in a blender and apply to skin folds and feet after washing to help prevent fungal infection.

HERBALISM

Phytotherapy – the use of plant extracts for healing – is one of the most exciting areas of medical research. Traditional herbs have provided orthodox medicine with many powerful drugs including aspirin (from the willow tree), digoxin (from the foxglove) and even potent new cancer treatments such as paclitaxel (from the Pacific Yew tree). World-wide, specialists known as ethnobiologists are continually seeking new products from among the traditional herbs used by native healers. The Amazon has proved to be one of the richest sources, providing a wide range of traditional remedies.

Different parts of different plants are used – roots, stems, flowers, leaves, bark, sap, fruit or seeds – depending on which has the highest concentration of active ingredient. In most cases these materials are dried and ground to produce a powder which is made into a tea, or packed into capsules for easy swallowing.

Aloe Vera

Aloe vera looks similar to a cactus but belongs to the lily family. There are many species of Aloe, or which four have medical uses. *Aloe barbadensis* (Aloe vera) is reputed to have the most useful medicinal properties.

Aloe gel is squeezed from the succulent leaves, which can grow to over 60 cm long. This gel contains a unique mix of vitamins, amino acids, enzymes and minerals which have been valued for their healing properties for over 6,000 years. When diluted to form a juice, the extract is said to increase energy and is widely used to help a wide range of illnesses. It contains substances that have several healing effects:

■ anti-inflammatory (anthraquinones and natural plant steroids)
■ hastens wound healing (fibroblast growth factor)
■ powerful antioxidants (vitamins C, E, betacarotene)
■ antiseptic (saponins and anthraquinones) against bacteria, viruses and fungi.

Aloe vera is helpful in the treatment of:
■ oral thrush
■ intestinal Candidiasis
■ heartburn
■ gastritis (inflammation of the stomach)
■ peptic ulcers
■ constipation
■ Irritable Bowel Syndrome (IBS)
■ Crohn's disease
■ colitis (inflammation of the colon)
■ diverticulitis
■ haemorrhoids (piles)
■ threadworms.

It is also widely used to help treat several skin conditions, arthritis, and ME.

Aloe vera juice can be made from fresh liquid extract (gel) or from powdered Aloe. The fresh gel has to be stabilized within hours of harvesting to prevent oxidation and deactivation. When selecting a product, aim for one made from 100 per cent pure Aloe vera. Its strength needs to be at least 40 per cent by volume (ideally approaching 95 per cent) to be effective. Also choose one that is made from Aloe liquid rather than powder. You may find it more palatable to choose a product containing a little natural fruit juice (for example grape, apple) to improve the flavour, although some people with Candida find that fruit juice makes their symptoms worse.

Some women using Aloe vera notice that it increases their menstrual flow. Aloe vera stimulates uterine contractions; for this reason it should not be used during pregnancy. Similarly, it should be avoided when breastfeeding as its active ingredients are excreted in breastmilk and can produce diarrhoea in the infant.

Dose

15–50 ml Aloe gel/juice per day. Start with a small dose (for example 1 teaspoon) and work up to around 1–2 tablespoons per day to find the dose that suits you best. Aloe has a powerful cathartic effect and taking too much will produce a brisk laxative response. Swill Aloe juice in the mouth to help oral thrush. Aloe gel can also be rubbed into skin ringworm lesions 3 times a day.

Echinacea (Purple Coneflower)

Echinacea, or Purple Coneflower, is known to boost the immune system and increase resistance to viral, fungal and bacterial infections. It is a traditional remedy used by Sioux Native Americans to treat blood poisoning, infections such as boils, and snake bite. It is used by herbalists to help prevent recurrent upper respiratory tract infections such as the common cold, laryngitis, tonsillitis or sinusitis, and to treat skin complaints. A tincture of Echinacea can be used as a mouthwash to treat and help to prevent recurrent oral thrush.

Dose

Capsules containing the powdered root (500 mg) or an infusion made from boiling 2 teaspoons Echinacea root in 200 ml water can be taken twice a day with meals, to complement the treatment of Candida infections. A tincture of Echinacea can be taken by mouth (4 ml) or applied undiluted to ringworm lesions 3 times a day.

Garlic (*Allium sativa*)

Garlic is a member of the Lily family. Its bulbs are divided into segments known as cloves. World-wide, each person eats an average of 1 clove garlic per day. The cloves contain a variety of volatile oils which have powerful antimicrobial actions. Garlic is effective against disease-causing bacteria, viruses and intestinal infections – including Candida – yet does not seem to harm beneficial intestinal bacteria such as *Lactobacillus*. Garlic can also be used externally to treat skin ringworm infections and warts, although some people develop a severe skin reaction – it is wise to protect surrounding skin with petroleum jelly and to wash the garlic juice off if the area becomes uncomfortable. The most common use of garlic is as a medication to lower blood pressure and reduce the risk of coronary heart disease.

Dose
Powdered garlic (in tablet form), 600–900 mg per day.

Ginseng

Siberian ginseng (*Eleutherococcus senticosus*) is used extensively to improve stamina and strength, particularly during or after illness. It seems to help the body adapt when under physical or emotional stress and can also boost immunity. When given to 13,000 workers at a Russian car factory, the number of days off work due to health problems dropped by a third. Siberian ginseng – and related roots such as Korean ginseng (*Panax ginseng*) and American ginseng (*Panax quinquefolium*) – are useful herbal supplements to take when you are feeling under the weather, or suffering from a relapse of symptoms that is dragging you down.

Dose
0.2 g–1 g, 3 times a day

Golden Seal

Golden Seal (*Hydrastis canadensis*) is an astringent anti-fungal herb whose roots are used to treat several skin conditions, including ringworm, eczema and itching (pruritis). It can stimulate immunity by increasing the activity of white blood cells. As Golden Seal also stimulates uterine contractions, it should be avoided during pregnancy.

Dose

An infusion of 1 teaspoon powdered root steeped in boiling water for 15 minutes can be cooled and used to soak ringworm lesions or Athlete's foot. Alternatively, the infusion can be applied directly to lesions 3 times a day. A tincture of Golden Seal can be taken by mouth (4 ml) or applied undiluted to ringworm lesions 3 times a day.

Guarana

Guarana comes from the Brazilian rain forest where it is known as the Food of the Gods. Sun-dried extracts from its seeds are used to make a sweet, cola-like, stimulating tonic containing a complex of natural stimulants similar to caffeine. It lifts the mood and stimulates the immune system but without the side-effects associated with drinking too much caffeine. The active ingredients, including guaranine, are buffered by special oils (saponins) to produce a natural time-release effect. A single dose of Guarana will provide a natural energy boost that lasts for up to 6 hours. Although it acts as a stimulant, it also has a calming effect and will not interfere with sleep or make stress-related symptoms worse. Research in Denmark found that after taking Guarana extracts for 3 months, volunteers had a significant increase in energy levels and reacted better to stress. As well as boosting the immune system, Guarana can thin the blood, reduce fluid retention and raise the metabolic rate.

Guarana is used to:

- relieve exhaustion and chronic fatigue
- increase mental alertness and concentration
- improve physical performance
- relieve stress
- help nervous insomnia
- relieve mild depression

- relieve tension headache and migraine
- relieve pre-menstrual syndrome and period pains
- hasten convalescence.

Dose

Guarana is available in capsules, a wine-based elixir, energy bars, as a chewing gum and in an energy drink. The recommended dose is 1 gram per day.

Lapacho

Lapacho is an unusual Brazilian tree with carnivorous flowers. These feed on insects, keeping it free from parasites and infections. Research in the US and Japan has found that extracts from Lapacho bark can stimulate the human immune system to increase resistance to infection, aid healing and reduce inflammatory reactions and pain. Its extracts are active against fungi including Candida, certain bacteria and malaria. Lapacho is used to treat a number of conditions, including:

- Candida (thrush)
- skin infections, including poorly healing wounds
- colds and other viral illnesses such as influenza
- boils
- urinary tract infections
- rheumatism and arthritis
- multiple sclerosis
- diabetes
- snake bite.

In Japan, a substance known as lapachol has been isolated from Lapacho and is currently being evaluated in trials to treat certain cancers.

Dose

A cup of Lapacho tea or 4 ml tincture can be taken daily to help prevent Candida infections. When treating an acute problem, doses can be increased by as much as 6 times. The infusion can also be used to bathe areas of infection such as ringworm, balanitis or vulvitis. Alternatively, take 1–2 g powdered bark by mouth in capsule form. (May cause nausea or diarrhoea if taken in very high doses.)

Marigold

Marigold petals have excellent anti-fungal properties. As well as being used internally and externally to treat infections such as Candida, Marigold is also used to help treat indigestion, peptic ulcers and gallbladder problems.

Dose
Pour 200 ml boiling water onto 2 teaspoons petals and infuse for 15 minutes. Drink 3 times a day. A tincture of Marigold (4 ml) can be taken by mouth or applied undiluted to ringworm lesions 3 times a day. Marigold can be combined with Golden Seal and Myrrh to make an anti-fungal wash.

Myrrh

Myrrh is a gum resin secreted by an East African bush. It stimulates the immune system by increasing the production of white blood cells and also has an antimicrobial effect. It is used as a mouthwash to treat mouth infections, including oral thrush, and is drunk to help combat infections such as boils, viral illnesses and Candida.

Dose
2 teaspoons powdered myrrh should be added to 200 ml boiling water and allowed to steep for 15 minutes. Cool and drink 3 times a day. A tincture of myrrh (4 ml) can be used as a mouthwash, applied undiluted to ringworm lesions or drunk 3 times a day.

Pfaffia

The golden root of *Pfaffia paniculata* is often referred to as the Brazilian ginseng, although it is unrelated to the Oriental varieties. Like the ginsengs, however, Pfaffia is a powerful 'adaptogen', which means it helps the body's immune system to adapt to various stresses including overwork, illness and fatigue. It is regarded as a panacea for all ills, as well as a sustaining food by local Brazilian Indians, who call it *para todo* – 'for everything'. It is a rich source of vitamins, minerals, amino acids and plant hormones (which act as building-blocks for the female hormone, oestrogen). It is therefore useful for treating gynaecological problems linked with hormonal imbalances such as pre-menstrual syndrome and menopausal symptoms. Because of its hormone content, Pfaffia should not be taken by pregnant women. Pfaffia is used to:

- boost energy levels
- improve physical and mental stamina
- increase concentration
- speed convalescence
- improve cellulite
- relieve pre-menstrual syndrome
- relieve menopausal symptoms
- help symptoms related to the oral contraceptive Pill
- relieve impotence
- relieve arthritis
- help maintain normal blood sugar levels in people with diabetes (use with medical supervision only).

Dose
1 gram per day.

Thuja

Thuja – the Tree of Life – is a member of the Cypress family. Its young twigs contain a volatile oil that tones muscles and is used in the treatment of cystitis, rheumatism and skin conditions such as psoriasis, ringworm or warts. As Thuja also causes uterine contractions, it should not be taken during pregnancy.

Dose
Pour 200 ml boiling water onto 1 teaspoon dried leaves and infuse for 15 minutes. Drink 3 times a day. A tincture of Thuja

(2 ml) can be taken by mouth or applied undiluted to ringworm lesions 3 times a day.

HOMOEOPATHY

Homoeopathic medicine is based on the belief that natural substances can boost the body's own healing powers to relieve the symptoms and signs of illness. Natural substances are selected which, if used full-strength in a healthy person, would produce symptoms of the illness they are designed to treat. This is the first principle of homoeopathy: 'Like cures Like.'

The second major principle of homoeopathy is that increasing the dilution of a solution has the opposite effect, that is, increases its potency ('Less Cures More'). By diluting noxious and even poisonous substances many millions of times, their healing properties are enhanced while their undesirable side-effects are lost.

On the centesimal scale, dilutions of 100^{-6} (1 drop tincture mixed with 99 drops alcohol or water and shaken; this is then done a further 6 times, each time 1 drop of the dilution being added to 99 drops of alcohol or water) are described as potencies of 6C, dilutions of 100^{-30} are written as a potency of 30C, etc. To illustrate just how diluted these substances are, a dilution of 12C (100^{-12}) is comparable to a pinch of salt dissolved in the same amount of water as is found in the Atlantic Ocean!

Homoeopathy is thought to work in a dynamic way, boosting your body's own healing powers. The principles behind homoeopathy may be difficult to accept, yet convincing trials have shown that homoeopathic therapy is significantly better than placebos in treating many chronic (long-term) conditions including hayfever, asthma and rheumatoid arthritis.

Homoeopathic remedies should ideally be taken on their own, at least 30 minutes either before or after eating or drinking. Tablets should not be handled – tip them into the lid of the container, or onto a teaspoon to transfer them into your mouth. Then suck or chew them, don't swallow them whole.

Homoeopathic treatments are prescribed according to your symptoms rather than any particular disease, so two people with the same label of 'Candidiasis' who have different symptoms will need different homoeopathic treatments. Two homoeopathic remedies in particular – Borax and Candida – have been shown in studies to be significantly more effective in treating symptoms of Candidiasis than placebo (inactive) substances. It is best to obtain individual professional advice before using these, however, as they are not indicated in every case.

Homoeopathic remedies may be prescribed by a medically-trained homoeopathic doctor on a normal NHS prescription form and dispensed by homoeopathic pharmacists for the usual prescription charge (or exemption, where applicable). Alternatively, you can consult a private homoeopathic practitioner or buy remedies direct from the pharmacist.

Although it is best to see a trained homoeopath who can assess your constitutional type, personality, lifestyle, family background, likes and dislikes as well as your symptoms before deciding which treatment is right for you, you may find the remedies listed below helpful. After taking the remedies for the time stated, if there is no obvious improvement consult a practitioner. Don't be surprised if your symptoms initially get worse before they get better – persevere through this common reaction to treatment – it is a good sign which shows the remedy is working.

- *Calc. carb 6C*: for vaginal Candida with a milky, itchy discharge, especially if linked with pre-menstrual symptoms, headache, stress, overwork or pregnancy. (6 times a day for up to 5 days)
- *Sepia 6C*: for vaginal Candida with an offensive discharge that is worse after making love, especially if linked with menstruation or the menopause. (6 times a day for up to 5 days)
- *Sulphur 6C*: for vaginal Candida with burning pains, especially if linked with stress or another illness (for example, one for which antibiotics were taken); for intestinal Candida linked with symptoms of alternating constipation and diarrhoea plus flatulence; for intestinal Candida linked with symptoms of anal itching or irritation around the anus. (6 times a day for up to 5 days)

Bach Rescue Remedy

This homoeopathic preparation is designed to help you cope with life's ups and downs and reduce the physical and emotional symptoms of stress and chronic illness such as recurrent Candida. It contains 5 flower essences: Cherry Plum, Clematis, Impatiens, Rock Rose and Star of Bethlehem, preserved in brandy. Add 4 drops of Rescue Remedy to a glass of water and sip slowly, every 3 to 5 minutes, holding the liquid in your mouth for a while before you swallow. Alternatively, place 4 drops directly under your tongue. Useful for acute recurrences of symptoms that leave you feeling unable to cope.

After completing a course of homoeopathy, you will usually feel much better in yourself with a greatly improved sense of well-being that helps you to cope with any remaining symptoms in a much more positive way.

Well-known naturopath Jan de Vries has also designed his own Emergency Essence, up-dated for modern times. This contains essences of Chamomile, Lavender, Red Clover, Purple Coneflower, Self-heal and Yarrow.

PROBIOTICS

Many patients have found that live yoghurt eaten every day relieves their symptoms. The Lactobacilli bacteria in live (Bio) yoghurt can happily line your bowel and keep it healthy and regular – they seem to survive the passage through stomach acids in enough numbers to recolonize the bowel. Use Bio yoghurt containing *Lactobacillus acidophilus*, eating at least 1 carton (150 ml) low-fat yoghurt per day. In addition, you may also benefit from a yoghurt-like liquid supplement (Yakult) containing a culture of *Lactobacillus casei* Shirota. This was developed by a team of scientists in Europe to replenish the bowel with a healthy, human strain of *Lactobacillus*.

Supplements are also available in health food shops containing *Lactobacillus acidophilus*, *Lactobacillus bulgaricus* and related species of beneficial bacteria such as *Bifidobacterium bifidum* and *Bifidobacterium longum*. These can be taken in powder/capsule form or used to make your own yoghurt cultures.

REFLEXOLOGY

This technique was used in China over 5,000 years ago and was also popular with the ancient Egyptians. Reflexology is based on the principle that points in the feet – known as reflexes – are directly related to other parts of the body. Massage over these reflexes can detect areas of tenderness and subtle textural changes which help to pinpoint problems in various organs, including the gut. By working on these tender spots with tiny pressure movements, nerves are thought to be stimulated that pass messages to distant organs, to relieve symptoms. Some people with Candida have found reflexology helpful.

SILICIC ACID

Silicon is one of the most common elements on Earth, coming second only to oxygen. It makes up 40 per cent of the Earth's crust and is found in a variety of substances including brick, cement, glass, quartz, emeralds, silicon chips and even non-stick frying pans. The foods with the richest content of silicon include wholegrain wheat, potatoes and unprocessed barley, oats, and rye.

Although silicon in its pure form is biologically inactive, it is now recognized as an essential trace element. In its soluble (colloidal) state, silicic acid, it is essential for normal growth and development. Silicic acid occurs naturally in low concentrations in most food and water. More and more people are now using colloidal silicic acid as a health supplement.

Colloidal silicic acid can be helpful in treating the symptoms of oral and intestinal Candida. It comes in the form of a gel which, when taken internally, reduces symptoms of bloating, flatulence and irregular bowel habit, especially diarrhoea. It has also proved helpful for more serious bowel problems such as ulcerative colitis and Crohn's disease.

As well as protecting the intestinal tract, silicic acid can soothe mouth ulcers and inflamed gums (gingivitis). It lines the stomach, absorbs toxins and irritants, and protects an inflamed stomach lining from self-digestion with stomach acid. It is therefore effective in the treatment of acid indigestion (gastritis) and heartburn due to acid reflux up into the gullet (reflux oesophagitis). It is safe to use during pregnancy.

Silicic acid should be taken in a dose of 1 tablespoon (30 ml) daily, diluted with fruit juice if preferred. Silicic acid gel can also be held and swirled in the mouth before swallowing to help relieve mouth soreness.

VISUALIZATION

When you feel symptoms of Candida getting on top of you, try visualization to aid relaxation and relieve your distress.

Stop what you are doing and sit down somewhere private and quiet. Close your eyes and, instead of focusing on your symptoms, imagine yourself:

- walking through a sunlit forest glade, with the sound of gently running water and bird song surrounding you, while a cool breeze ruffles your hair
- swimming in a warm tropical ocean next to a white-sand, deserted beach
- sitting in the sun on the veranda of a log chalet high up on a snow-crested mountain – breathe in the cool air and hear the soft drip of snow melting from the surrounding fir trees.

Visualization has been shown to help bowel problems including inflammatory bowel disease and Irritable Bowel Syndrome, as well as aiding relaxation.

Chapter Ten

CANDIDA AND YOUR DIET

CANDIDA AND DIETARY DEFICIENCIES

It is estimated that only 1 in 10 people gets all the necessary essential fatty acids, vitamins and minerals from diet alone. As chronic (long-term) or recurrent Candida is linked with a faulty immune system, many researchers believe that lack of dietary nutrients is linked with an increased risk of developing symptoms.

Vitamins, minerals and essential fatty acids in your food are all needed for:

- healthy cell membranes and skin
- making the enzymes used in fighting infections
- as co-factors to help enzyme function
- making the chemicals that enable immune cells to communicate with one another
- making substances involved in inflammation
- proper healing.

Even if only one nutrient is in short supply (for example iron) it may be enough to tip the balance in favour of yeast overgrowth. At the same time, Candida yeasts cells also need nutrients to grow and put out germ tubes (hyphae) as they start to invade tissues. It is therefore important that your diet and intake of nutrients are balanced. If taking a vitamin and mineral supplement, for example, it is best to take one that supplies around 100 per cent of the recommended daily amount (RDA) of as many vitamins and minerals as possible.

Evening Primrose Oil

The beautiful Evening Primrose flower only blooms for a single day, but a valuable oil can be extracted from its seeds to provide one of the most popular and useful food supplements available. It can help a wide range of problems, from dry itchy skin, eczema, psoriasis and acne to pre-menstrual syndrome, menopausal problems and cyclical breast pain. It has also proved useful in the treatment of Irritable Bowel Syndrome (IBS), rheumatoid arthritis, high cholesterol levels and high blood pressure. It is also an immune stimulant and improves resistance to infections, as well as being under investigation for its anti-cancer properties.

Evening Primrose Oil is a rich source of an essential fatty acid (EFA) called GLA (gamma linolenic acid – sometimes shortened to gamolenic acid). These essential fatty acids cannot be made in the body in sufficient amounts to meet your needs and must therefore come from your diet. There are three essential fatty acids:

1. linolenic acid (of which one type is gamma-linolenic acid)
2. linoleic acid
3. arachidonic acid (can be synthesized from linolenic or linoleic acids).

THE EFA PATHWAY

Linoleic acid → Gamma-linolenic acid (GLA) (Evening Primrose Oil) → dihomo-gamma linolenic acid → arachidonic acid → prostaglandins

Essential fatty acids, including GLA, are metabolized in the body to form hormone-like substances known as prostaglandins. Prostaglandins are found in all body tissues and play a major role in regulating inflammation, blood clotting and hormone balance, and are involved in the immune responses concerned with infections, chronic inflammatory diseases and even cancer. Nutritional deficiency of EFAs is common. While the body can make do with other fatty acids in their place (for example saturated animal fatty acids) this results in prostaglandin imbalances, as those made from other sorts of fat cannot be converted into prostaglandins. This imbalance is thought to increase the risk of developing:

- cell membranes that are stiffer than normal
- dry, itchy, flaky skin, which increases the risk of Candida infections taking hold
- inflammatory diseases
- blood clots
- lowered immunity against infections such as Candida
- hormone imbalances.

If your diet is lacking in GLA, gamma-linolenic acid can be synthesized from dietary linoleic acid, but this reaction relies on a particular enzyme (delta-6-desaturase) that is easily blocked by a number of factors, including:

- eating too much saturated (animal) fat
- eating too many trans-fatty acids (for example those found in margarines)
- eating too much sugar
- drinking too much alcohol
- deficiency of vitamins and minerals, especially vitamin B$_6$, zinc and magnesium
- increasing age
- crash dieting
- smoking cigarettes
- exposure to pollution.

Taking Evening Primrose Oil supplements provides dietary GLA and feeds into the EFA pathway, bypassing any enzyme blocks and helping to correct any prostaglandin or hormone imbalances. It is so effective that doctors can prescribe Evening Primrose Oil to treat eczema and mastalgia (cyclical breast pain).

Many people find that taking an Evening Primrose Oil supplement helps to break their recurrent Candida cycle as it provides important building-blocks for immune cells and protective immune reactions.

When choosing an Evening Primrose Oil (EPO) supplement:

- Select one containing 100 per cent pure EPO.
- Choose one containing at least 500 mg EPO per capsule plus some vitamin E, which helps to protect the GLA content from oxidation and boosts its function.
- Certain vitamins and minerals are needed during the metabolism of essential fatty acids. These are vitamin C, vitamin B_6, vitamin B_3 (niacin), zinc and magnesium. If you are taking EPO, make sure your intake of these is also adequate.

For general preventive health, take 500–1,000 mg EPO per day.

For treating a specific condition, you may need to take 3,000–4,000 mg per day for at least 3 months to correct a long-term imbalance, before you can tell if it is producing a beneficial effect.

Taking too much EPO may cause mild diarrhoea. Some women taking high-dose supplements have noticed breast enlargement or a change in their normal period pattern, but these side-effects are not usually too troublesome.

If you suffer from temporal lobe epilepsy (an uncommon nervous disorder), only take EPO under medical supervision.

Some evidence suggests that EPO supplement are best taken late in the afternoon (between 4 and 6 p.m.).

DIETARY SOURCES OF ESSENTIAL FATTY ACIDS

- Linoleic acid is found in sunflower seeds, almonds, corn, sesame seeds, safflower oil and extra virgin olive oil.
- Linolenic acid is found in Evening Primrose Oil, starflower (borage) seed oil and blackcurrant seed oil.
- Both linoleic and linolenic acids are found in rich quantities in walnuts, pumpkin seeds, soybeans, linseed oil, rapeseed oil and flax oil.
- Arachidonic acid is found in many foods (for example seafood, meat, dairy products) and can also be made from linoleic or linolenic acids.

Vitamin and Mineral Deficiencies

Vitamins are naturally occurring organic substances which, although they are only needed in minute amounts, are essential for life. They cannot be synthesized in the body, or if they can (for example vitamin D, niacin) are made in amounts too small to meet your needs. They must therefore come from your food. Most vitamins act as essential intermediaries or catalysts to keep metabolic reactions running smoothly and efficiently. These reactions include:

■ converting fats and carbohydrates into energy
■ digestion of foods
■ cell division and growth
■ repair of damaged tissues
■ healthy blood
■ fighting infection
■ mental alertness
■ healthy reproduction
■ mopping up harmful by-products of metabolism such as free radicals.

Minerals are inorganic elements, some of which are metals, which are essential for metabolic reactions. Those needed in amounts of less than 100 mg are often referred to as trace elements. Minerals and trace elements can only come from your diet and depend on the quality of soil on which produce is grown or grazed. Minerals have a number of functions:

■ structural – for example, calcium, magnesium and phosphate strengthen bones and teeth
■ maintenance – for example, sodium, potassium, calcium support normal cell function
■ as co-factors for important enzymes – for example, copper, iron, magnesium, manganese, molybdenum, selenium, zinc
■ involvement in oxygen transport – for example, iron
■ regulation of hormone function – for example, chromium, iodine
■ antioxidant – for example, selenium, manganese.

Some trace elements such as nickel, tin and vanadium are known to be essential for normal growth in only tiny amounts, although their exact roles are not yet fully understood.

Minor vitamin and mineral deficiencies are common. Lack of nutrients is rarely severe enough to cause the sort of deficiency diseases seen in the third world (for example scurvy, beri-beri) but they can be enough to impair your immunity and increase your risk of a number of diseases, including Candida. For example:

- 60 per cent of the population does not obtain the new EC recommended daily amounts (RDA) of 60 mg vitamin C on a regular basis
- 90 per cent of the population does not obtain the recommended 10 mg vitamin E.
- 99 per cent of people obtain less than 2 mg betacarotene per day from their food – the National Cancer Institute in the US suggests a minimum intake of 6 mg betacarotene per day (equivalent to 100 ml carrot juice) to protect against cancer.
- Average intakes of vitamin B_1 and B_2 are below recommended levels.
- 50 per cent of adults obtain less vitamin B_6 than ideal.

The situation with minerals is even worse. The 1993 UK Government Food Survey shows that a large proportion of the population is at risk of gross deficiency in 8 out of 13 vitamins and minerals. Compared with the new EC RDAs, the average adult only obtains:

- 53 per cent of the RDA for zinc
- 56 per cent of the RDA for vitamin D
- 68 per cent of the RDA for iron
- 78 per cent of the RDA for magnesium

and 40 per cent of people obtained less dietary calcium than recommended.

Another Government report confirms that the average intake of the mineral selenium has fallen dramatically, from 60 mcg in 1978 to just 34 mcg in 1995. The ideal intakes are 75 mcg for men and 60 mcg for women.

Even when the lowest possible intake of a mineral – the amount necessary to prevent deficiency disease – is measured, one UK Government survey found:

PROPORTION OF WOMEN WITH INTAKES BELOW THE LOWER REFERENCE NUTRIENT INTAKE (LRNI)

Nutrient	16–18 years LRNI/ %	19–50 years LRNI/ %	51–64 years LRNI/ %
Calcium (mg)	480/27 %	400/10 %	400/5 %
Iron (mg)	8/33 %	8/26 %	8/1 %
Magnesium (mg)	190/39 %	150/13 %	150/9 %
Potassium (mg)	2000/30 %	2000/27 %	2000/23 %

Dietary and Nutritional Survey of British Adults – Further Analysis MAFF. HMSO

And that's just for the lower reference nutrient intake. When you consider that optimum intakes of calcium are at least 800 mg per day, and that menstruating women ideally need at least 14 mg iron per day the number of women obtaining less than optimal levels of minerals is frightening. The recommended intakes that will supply the needs of at least 96 per cent of the population are:

VITAMIN	RDA
Vitamin A (retinol)	800 mcg
Vitamin B_1 (thiamin)	1.4 mg
Vitamin B_2 (riboflavin)	1.6 mg
Vitamin B_3 (niacin)	18 mg
Vitamin B_5 (pantothenic acid)	6 mg
Vitamin B_6 (pyridoxine)	2 mg
Vitamin B_{12} (cyanocobalamin)	1 mcg
Biotin	0.15 mg
Folic Acid	200 mcg
Vitamin C	60 mg
Vitamin D	5 mcg
Vitamin E	10 mg

MINERAL

Calcium	800 mg
Iodine	150 mcg
Iron	14 mg
Magnesium	300 mg
Phosphorus	800 mg
Zinc	15 mg

Lack of vitamins and minerals can cause a number of common symptoms, including:

- lowered immunity
- recurrent infections
- poor wound healing
- feeling tired all the time
- mouth ulcers
- sore tongue
- cracked lips
- inflamed gums
- scaly skin
- brittle nails and hair
- pre-menstrual syndrome
- constipation
- nerve conduction problems
- muscle weakness.

Why Your Diet may be Poor in Vitamins and Minerals

Many people feel they are already following a healthy diet and are unlikely to be lacking in vitamins and minerals – but you are totally reliant upon the quality and age of your food, as well as the way it has been stored and processed. Even if crops leave the soil with a good nutrient content, processing can strip much of this out:

- Food staples are grown in artificially fertilized soils boosted with nitrogen, phosphorus and potassium. Other minerals and trace elements are frequently depleted. This may not interfere with plant growth, but seriously reduces the nutritional benefit to you.

- Fruit and vegetables are bred for uniformity of colour and shape rather than for flavour and nutrient content.
- Pesticides and other pollutants interfere with the nutrient content of plants.
- Foods are heavily processed or pre-packaged for convenience.
- Foods are shipped from abroad and may be picked before they are ripe – nutrient content falls as a result.
- Food additives interfere with the nutrient content of prepared foods.
- Stored foods rapidly lose their vitamin content.
- Cooking foods rather than eating them raw decreases their nutrient content – either by destroying it or leaching it into the cooking water.
- Wholefoods are eaten less frequently – we prefer to eat more animal and dairy foods, which are full of saturated fats.
- We now eat more trans-fatty acids – chemicals which interfere with the way our body metabolizes micronutrients and essential fatty acids.
- Mechanical and chemical food processing is the biggest cause of poor nutrient intakes.

Mechanical and chemical food processing is perhaps one of the biggest causes of our nutritionally poor Western diet. Processing strips formerly nutritious foods of their vitamin and mineral content.

Vitamin A
- Boiling or frying reduces the vitamin A content of food by 40 per cent after 1 hour – and by 70 per cent after 2 hours (for example in the slow cooking of stews).
- Canning vegetables depletes them of 20–35 per cent of their vitamin A.
- Drying fruit and vegetables results in the loss of up to 20 per cent – open-air drying in the loss of all vitamin A activity.

Vitamin B_1 (thiamin)
- A common preservative in minced meat (sulphur dioxide) destroys 90 per cent of a food's thiamin content within 2 days.

- Up to 70 per cent of a food's thiamin content is lost into cooking juices if food is finely chopped or minced.
- Cooking meat at 200°C causes a further 20 per cent destruction of thiamin content.
- Baking (for example in bread) reduces thiamin content by up to 30 per cent.
- Adding baking powder increases losses to 50 per cent.
- Toasting bread reduces thiamin by a further 10–30 per cent.
- Additives used to keep processed potatoes white (sulphite) reduce their thiamin content by over 50 per cent.
- Freezing meats reduces their thiamin content by up to 50 per cent.

Vitamins B_2 (riboflavin) and B_3 (niacin)

- Light is the most usual destroyer of B_2 – 90 per cent is lost from milk after only 2 hours' sun exposure.
- Boiling milk reduces its riboflavin content by up to 25 per cent.
- Curing meats reduces vitamin B_3 content by up to 40 per cent
- Freezing meats reduces riboflavin by up to 50 per cent.
- Riboflavin is also readily lost into cooking water.

Vitamin B_5 (pantothenic acid)

- Processing wheat can reduce its content of vitamin B_5 by 60 per cent.
- 30 per cent of the vitamin B_5 in meat is lost into cooking juices.
- Freezing causes a slow destruction of this vitamin.

Vitamin B_6 (pyridoxine)

- 20 per cent of the vitamin B_6 in milk is destroyed by sterilization.
- 20 per cent in vegetables is lost by canning.
- 40 per cent is lost into water when frozen vegetables are thawed and cooked.
- Up to 70 per cent of vitamin B_6 in meat is lost during processing.

Vitamin B$_{12}$
- Around 20 per cent is leached into water during cooking.

Folate
- Up to 90 per cent of the folate content of grain is lost during milling.
- 10 per cent of the folate in vegetables is lost by steaming, 20 per cent by pressure-cooking and up to 50 per cent by boiling.
- Foods originally rich in folate may have less than one-third of their folate content left by the time they are eaten.

Vitamin C
- Processing soft fruits (for example berries) results in the loss of over two-thirds of their vitamin C content.
- Once fruit juices are opened, their vitamin C content rapidly deteriorates, even if chilled – virtually all is lost within 14 days.
- Boiling vegetables leaves behind up to 50 per cent of vitamin C into the cooking water.
- Storage of root vegetables (for example potatoes) robs them of around 10 per cent of their vitamin C content per month.
- Storage of some vegetables (for example asparagus) reduces their vitamin C content by up to 90 per cent after just 1 week.

Vitamin E
- This vitamin is rapidly depleted by exposure to air.
- Even when frozen, foods can lose up to 70 per cent of their vitamin E content within 14 days.
- Processing cereals and grains removes over 90 per cent of their vitamin E content (for example in the production of white flour).
- Cooking foods in fat (for example frying or roasting) will destroy virtually all their vitamin E content, especially if the oils are rancid (for example if you re-use fat in a chip fryer for too long).
- Boiling exhausts a third of the vitamin E content of vegetables.
- Canning methods increase losses by up to 80 per cent.

Magnesium
- 80 per cent of the magnesium in wholegrains is lost during milling.

Obtaining Maximum Goodness from Your Food

- Eat food as fresh as possible – preferably home or locally grown.
- Eat foods grown using organic farming methods where possible – these are usually significantly more expensive weight for weight, but not when measured in nutrients per pound.
- Avoid processed, pre-packaged convenience foods.
- Eat as many raw fruits and vegetables as possible.
- Eat more wholegrains, nuts and seeds.
- Cook fruit and vegetables as little as possible. Steam vegetables lightly or use only a small amount of water when boiling.
- Re-use juices from cooking vegetables, for example in sauces, soups or gravy.

Increasing numbers of experts now believe that taking a food supplement is essential for optimal health. Although there is no guarantee that this will improve your Candida symptoms, it will certainly guard against the common nutrient deficiencies and help to optimize your overall health. It may also prevent some of the common, niggling health problems linked with mild vitamin and mineral deficiency.

Important Vitamins and Minerals for Candida Sufferers

The vitamins and minerals thought to be most beneficial in overcoming Candida infections are the B group vitamins, antioxidants (vitamins C, E and betacarotene) and the minerals iron, selenium and zinc. Make sure any supplement you take includes these in sensible amounts, and ensure that you eat plenty of foods that are rich sources of them.

Betacarotene
Betacarotene is made up of 2 molecules of vitamin A joined together. It is converted into vitamin A in the body when needed

(6 mcg betacarotene = around 1 mcg of vitamin A [retinol]). Zinc is essential for this conversion. On average, around half of the betacarotene in your diet is converted into vitamin A in the cells lining the small intestine and in your liver. It is needed to:

- regulate the way genes are 'read' to produce enzymes and other proteins
- control normal growth and development, sexual health and reproduction
- maintain healthy skin, teeth, bones and mucous membranes such as those found lining the nose, throat and gums
- produce the pigment known as visual purple (rhodopsin), which is involved in sight and night vision.

Lack of betacarotene/vitamin A can cause:
- increased susceptibility to infections such as Candida
- scaly skin with raised, pimply hair follicles that encourage fungal skin infections
- flaking scalp
- brittle, dull hair
- poor eyesight and night vision
- loss of appetite
- loss of sensitivity to green light and difficulty adapting to dim light
- dry, burning, itchy eyes – and in the extreme, eye ulceration
- inflamed gums and mucous membranes.

Daily intakes of betacarotene above 15 mg per day may turn skin a yellow-orange colour – this looks like an artificial tan but is not harmful. High intakes in smokers have been linked with an increased risk of lung cancer. Betacarotene is best taken along with other antioxidants such as vitamin E and vitamins C.

Good food sources of betacarotene:
Dark green leafy vegetables and yellow-orange fruits, for example:

- carrots
- sweet potatoes

- spinach
- broccoli
- parsley
- spinach
- watercress
- spring greens
- cantaloupe melons
- apricots
- peaches
- mango
- red-yellow peppers
- tomatoes
- sweet corn.

Vitamin A is easily destroyed by exposure to light. Betacarotene is destroyed by heat and overcooking.

Vitamin B Group
- Vitamin B_1 (thiamin)
- Vitamin B_2 (riboflavin)
- Vitamin B_3 (niacin)
- Vitamin B_5 (pantothenic acid)
- Vitamin B_6 (pyridoxine)
- Vitamin B_{12} (cobalamin)
- Folic acid
- Biotin

The B group vitamins have a number of important functions in the body. Some are made by intestinal micro-organisms such as bacteria and yeasts – when there is a dietary deficiency, they may compete for your supplies. Bowel bacteria usually make lots of biotin, which you can absorb so that deficiency is rare unless you eat lots of raw egg white (for example sportsmen when training). Raw egg white contains a protein, avidin, that binds to biotin in the gut and prevents it from being absorbed. Cooked egg white does not have this effect. Interestingly, research suggests that biotin inhibits Candida growth and prevents it converting from a simple colonizing cell to the invasive mycelia form with germ tubes. It may be that people who are prone to intestinal Candida have bowel bacteria which do not produce as much biotin as usual.

B group vitamins are needed to:
- co-ordinate nerve and muscle cell functions
- produce energy from blood sugar (glucose) and fatty acids
- produce healthy red blood cells – lack of folate or vitamin B_{12} leads to anaemia
- for the healthy growth and division of cells – including in a developing fetus, where lack of folate and vitamin B_{12} are linked with congenital abnormalities such as Spina Bifida
- for the synthesis of amino acids.

Lack of B group vitamins can cause:
- tiredness
- pallor (anaemia)
- headache
- bloodshot, red eyes
- sores and cracks at the corner of the mouth
- red, inflamed tongue and lips
- mouth ulcers
- a scaly eczema-like skin rash, especially on the face and nose
- loss of appetite
- nausea
- constipation
- irritability
- loss of concentration
- poor memory
- difficulty sleeping
- difficulty coping with stress
- depression
- muscle weakness and stiffness
- nerve tingling, burning and numbness.

Large doses of niacin (B_3) may cause flushing and can lead to nausea, headache, muscle cramps, diarrhoea, low blood pressure. Very high doses are toxic and can cause liver damage. Excess B_6 (over 100 mg per day) may lead to reversible nerve damage (tingling, burning, shooting pains, pins and needles) and even partial paralysis.

Folic acid supplements can interfere with anti-epilepsy medication.

Good food sources of the B group vitamins include:
- brewer's yeast and yeast extracts (you may want to avoid these if you have Candida problems, however)
- brown rice
- wheat germ and wheat bran
- wholegrain bread and cereals
- oatmeal and oatflakes
- soya flour
- pasta
- meat and offal
- milk and dairy products
- seafood
- green leafy vegetables
- beans
- nuts.

Vitamin C

Vitamin C is a powerful antioxidant that helps to mop up harmful by-products of metabolism known as free radicals. By doing this, antioxidants help to damp down inflammatory reactions which are linked with long-term chronic illnesses such as Candida, rheumatism and colitis. It is also a natural antihistamine and helps to damp down allergic reactions. It has been shown to boost immunity, enhance the activity of white blood cells and reduce your risk of developing symptoms if you are exposed to the common cold virus and Candida. Vitamin C is also needed for:

- the synthesis of collagen, a major structural protein in the body
- the growth, repair and health of skin, bones, teeth and reproduction
- the metabolism of stress hormones.

Lack of vitamin C can cause:
- dry, rough, scaly skin
- scalp dryness
- hair loss
- broken thread veins in the skin
- poor wound healing
- misshapen, tangled, brittle hair
- dry, fissured lips
- easy bruising
- loose teeth
- inflamed, bleeding gums
- bleeding skin, eyes and nose
- weakness
- muscle and joint pain
- irritability
- depression.

Good food sources of vitamin C include:
- blackcurrants
- guavas
- kiwi fruit
- citrus fruit
- mangoes
- green peppers
- strawberries
- green sprouting vegetables such as broccoli, sprouts, watercress, parsley
- potatoes.

Vitamin E
Vitamin E is another powerful antioxidant which works mainly in the fatty tissues of your body where it is difficult for vitamin C to penetrate. It helps to:

- protect your cell membranes and body fat stores
- prevent dietary fats from going rancid
- strengthen muscle fibres
- improve skin suppleness and healing
- boost immunity.

Vitamin E is important for healing and works closely with the mineral, selenium, to boost immunity. Vitamins E and C should be taken together in supplement form, as once vitamin E has acted as an antioxidant, it needs vitamin C to reactivate it again.

Lack of vitamin E can cause:
- tiredness
- lethargy
- poor concentration
- irritability
- lowered sex drive
- muscle weakness.

Good food sources of vitamin E include:
- wheatgerm oil
- avocados
- margarine
- eggs
- butter
- wholemeal cereals
- seeds
- nuts
- bread
- oily fish
- broccoli.

Iron

Lack of iron is common, especially in women with a tendency towards heavy periods. This is because a large portion of the body's iron stores are in the form of the red blood pigment, haemoglobin, which transports oxygen and the waste gas, carbon dioxide, around the body. While long-term lack of iron can lead to anaemia, a mild shortage can increase your risk of infections. This is because blood stores of other iron-containing proteins (such as ferritin) are lowered. These proteins are needed by white blood cells to make the powerful chemicals used to kill invading micro-organisms. Lack of iron has been linked with an increased risk of recurrent Candidiasis and Herpes simplex virus infections. Iron is also:

- found in a protein, myoglobin, which binds oxygen in muscle cells
- a co-factor in many reactions involving energy production and immunity.

Lack of iron can cause:
- tiredness
- sore tongue
- cracking at the corners of the mouth
- decreased appetite
- increased susceptibility to infection
- generalized skin itching
- concave, brittle nails
- brittle hair and hair loss
- pallor (anaemia)
- muscle fatigue
- dizziness
- headache
- insomnia.

Good food sources of iron include:
- shellfish
- brewer's yeast
- offal (liver, kidney, heart)
- red meat
- fish, especially sardines
- wheatgerm
- wholemeal bread
- cocoa powder
- egg yolk
- green vegetables
- parsley
- prunes and other dried fruit

Selenium

Selenium is a mineral with a powerful antioxidant action. As well as damping down inflammatory reactions, it is needed for the synthesis of hormone-like prostaglandins and for the production of antibodies. Research suggests that antibody synthesis increases up to 30-fold if supplements of selenium and vitamin E – which work together – are taken. Selenium is also essential for healthy cell growth and division. People with the lowest intakes of selenium seem to have the highest risk of developing leukaemia or cancers of the colon, rectum, breast, ovary, pancreas, prostate gland, bladder, skin and lungs. These risks are even higher if intakes of vitamin E and vitamin A are also low.

Lack of selenium can cause:
- poor growth
- increased risk of infection
- hair, nail and skin problems
- premature wrinkling of skin
- subfertility
- arthritis
- high blood pressure
- cataracts
- muscle weakness
- Keshan disease (a form of heart failure).

Good food sources of selenium include:
- broccoli
- mushrooms
- cabbage
- radishes
- onions
- garlic
- celery
- wholegrains
- nuts
- brewer's yeast
- seafood
- offal
- butter.

Zinc

Zinc is essential for the proper function of over a hundred different enzymes, including many involved in immunity and fighting off infections such as Candida. It works by regulating the activation of genes as and when they are needed to make specific proteins such as antibodies. It is vital for growth, sexual maturity, wound healing and immune function.

One of the earliest symptoms of zinc deficiency is loss of your sense of taste. This can be tested for by obtaining a solution of zinc sulphate (5 mg/5 ml) from a chemist. Swirl a teaspoonful in your mouth. If the solution seems tasteless, zinc deficiency is likely. If the solution tastes furry, of minerals or slightly sweet, your zinc levels are borderline. If it tastes strongly unpleasant, your zinc levels are normal.

Lack of zinc may cause:
- impaired immunity and increased risk of infection
- poor wound healing
- poor hair growth and hair loss
- poor nail growth
- white spots on nails
- skin problems such as eczema, psoriasis, acne
- loss of your senses of taste and smell
- poor growth and delayed puberty
- underdeveloped male sex organs and low sperm count
- poor appetite
- cravings for odd foods
- diarrhoea
- visual disturbances
- mental sluggishness
- sleep disturbances.

If taken in doses larger than 15 mg, zinc may cause stomach upsets and nausea.

Good food sources of zinc include:
- red meat
- seafood, especially oysters
- offal
- brewer's yeast
- whole grains
- pulses

- eggs
- cheese.

Boosting Your Immune System

To boost your immune system without sticking to a strict anti-Candida regime:

- Follow a wholefood diet containing plenty of fresh fruit, vegetables and wholegrains with as few processed foods and additives as possible.
- Cut back on your intake of omega-6 polyunsaturated vegetable fats (found in margarine, cakes, biscuits, etc.) and eat more omega-3 essential fatty acids (such as those found in oily fish).
- Take a good vitamin and mineral supplement providing as many vitamins and minerals as possible at around 100 per cent of their recommended daily amount (RDA).
- Consider taking higher doses of the antioxidant vitamins C and E.
- Consider taking pure Evening Primrose Oil supplements.
- If you are zinc deficient, take 10 mg zinc twice a day for 2 weeks, then test yourself using a zinc sulphate solution (*see above*).
- If you smoke, stop.
- Limit your alcohol intake to no more than 1–2 units per day.
- Take regular exercise.
- Obtain adequate rest and sleep.

THE ANTI-CANDIDA DIET

Although some people view the anti-Candida diet with suspicion, it has undoubtedly helped many people with symptoms thought to be due to Candidiasis. There is little to lose by following an anti-Candida regime for a few weeks to see if it helps you. Trial and error are needed before you can isolate which foods bring your symptoms on, and the type of diet that keeps problems at bay. (For information on the types of food known to contain Candida cells, *see Chapter 6, page 72.*)

The basic anti-Candida diet involves avoiding products containing brewer's or baker's yeast, and products that stimulate yeast growth, including:

- white or brown sugar and food or drinks containing them (for example honey, jam, desserts, treacle, syrups, cakes, biscuits, sauces, ice-cream, soft drinks, dried fruits, chocolates, malt, etc.)
- refined (processed) carbohydrates (for example white flour, white rice) and products made from them (for example biscuits, cakes, buns, white bread)
- yeast extracts, cheese, bread made with yeast, alcoholic drinks, vinegar and pickled foods, smoked foods, soy sauce, tofu, grapes and grape juice, unpeeled fruits, dried fruits, frozen or concentrated fruit juices, old potentially mouldy foods and vegetables, mushrooms, and B vitamin supplements that are not labelled as 'yeast-free'
- some sugar substitutes such as sorbitol, mannitol, xylitol, aspartame and saccharin, which are metabolized like alcohol to produce substances that can stimulate Candida growth
- alcohol, tea, coffee, cocoa products, malted night-time drinks, fizzy drinks, fruit squashes.

It may take a few days for a change in diet to affect your symptoms. If you feel there is a definite link with a particular food, keep re-introducing it after avoiding it for several days to confirm that the effect is consistent. If you are fairly confident there is a problem, discuss this with your doctor or a dietitian to ensure that avoiding that particular food is not going to cause lack of any important nutrients – this is especially important if you are not overweight and find you start losing more than 1 or 2 pounds by following an anti-Candida programme.

If your symptoms are not significantly improved by following a restricted diet, it is important to return to eating a normal diet and as wide a range of foods as possible, to guard against any nutrient deficiencies. If you are able to identify a small number of foods which undoubtedly provoke your symptoms, however, these can usually be avoided without affecting your overall nutrition.

Other dietary measures to take include eating more:

- foods that tend to contain natural anti-fungal agents (for example garlic, herbs and spices, fresh green leafy vegetables)
- fibre-rich foods such as pulses (for example peas, beans, lentils, chick-peas) and wholegrain cereals (such as oats, brown rice, wholewheat pasta, whole rye, buckwheat, millet, bulgar wheat, couscous, unsweetened wholegrain breakfast cereals – but avoid those containing processed grains). In an ultra-strict anti-Candida diet, intakes of unrefined complex carbohydrates such as brown rice, wholegrain cereals and wholewheat pasta are also restricted (for example to the equivalent of just 2–3 slices wholegrain bread per day). As unrefined complex carbohydrates are an important part of a normal healthy diet, it is best not to follow a diet restricting these for more than 1 or 2 weeks without first taking expert dietary advice.
- more nuts and seeds for essential fatty acids (*see page 141*)
- fish
- raw or lightly steamed vegetables
- well-washed, peeled fruit
- extra virgin olive oil
- dairy products (an ultra-strict anti-Candida regime may ban these)
- natural BIO yoghurt and yoghurt-like drinks (for example Yakult) containing beneficial bacteria.

You should also drink plenty of mineral water and consider taking supplements containing:

- multivitamins and minerals – preferably providing around 100 per cent of the recommended daily amount (RDA) for as many vitamins and minerals as possible (check it does not contain yeast products)
- Evening Primrose Oil
- perhaps a supplement containing caprylic acid (*see below*).

Fibre

For every gram of fibre in your diet, your bowel motions increase by around 5 grams in weight. This is because dietary fibre provides nutrients for bacterial growth; much of the increased bowel motion bulk provided by a high-fibre diet is due to increased bacterial multiplication in the gut. This helps to keep intestinal Candida in check. Fibre also absorbs water and toxins (including yeast chemicals) from the gut, and helps to scour yeast cells from the intestinal wall, hastening their expulsion.

Fibre is an essential component of all plant cell structures. There are two main types of fibre: soluble and insoluble.

Soluble fibre is important in the stomach and upper intestines, where it slows down the processes of digestion and absorption. Blood sugar and fat levels only rise slowly, rather than rapidly, so the body can handle nutrient fluctuations more easily and there is less sugar available to encourage Candida growth.

Insoluble fibre is most important in the large bowel. It bulks up the faeces, absorbs water and hastens stool excretion.

All plant foods contain both soluble and insoluble fibre, though some sources are richer in one type than another. The following table gives some common examples of foods rich in dietary fibre:

SOURCES OF SOLUBLE AND INSOLUBLE FIBRE

Classification	Plant Source	A Few Examples
SOLUBLE		
	Oats	porridge, muesli
	Barley	pearl barley
	Rye	rye bread, crispbread
	Fruit	figs, apricots, tomatoes, apples
	Vegetables	carrots, potatoes, courgettes
	Pulses	cannellini beans, kidney beans

INSOLUBLE

Wheat	wholemeal bread, cereals
Maize	sweetcorn, corn bread
Rice	brown rice
Pasta	wholemeal pasta, spinach pasta
Fruit	rhubarb, blackberries, strawberries
Vegetables	cabbage, spinach, lettuce
Pulses	peas, lentils, chick peas

Ideally, you need to eat around 30 g fibre per day. Although this roughage provides little in the way of energy or nutrients, it is essential for helping the digestion and absorption of other foods. Fibre encourages the muscular, wave-like bowel contractions (peristalsis) that propel digested food through the intestines. This regulates bowel function and also acts like a sponge to absorb water, toxins, yeast cells and bacteria.

Research also suggests that dietary fibre absorbs fats and sugars in the bowel and helps to lower blood glucose and cholesterol levels by increasing the amount of fat that is excreted rather than absorbed.

A high-fibre diet helps to prevent constipation, diverticular disease, IBS and some bowel tumours – and may help reduce the symptoms associated with Candida. The easiest way to increase the amount of fibre in your diet is to eat more unrefined complex carbohydrates, as found in foods such as wholemeal bread, cereals, nuts, grains, root vegetables and fruits (unless following a strict anti-Candida regime, *see page 159*).

GRAMS OF FIBRE PER 100 G

- bran: 40 g fibre
- dried apricots: 18 g
- peas: 5 g
- prunes: 13 g
- cooked brown rice: 4 g
- cooked wholemeal spaghetti: 4 g
- brown bread: 6 g
- walnuts: 6 g

Breakfast Cereals Rich in Fibre

Bran-containing breakfast cereals provide the highest concentration of dietary fibre. There are many varieties available, including:

- muesli
- Bran Buds
- All Bran
- Bran Flakes
- Weetabix
- Puffed Wheat
- Shredded Wheat.

Caprylic Acid

Caprylic acid is a natural fatty acid found in coconut oil, palm oil and breastmilk. It has a natural anti-fungal action which has been shown to help eradicate *Candida albicans* from the gut without affecting the normal bacterial population. As caprylic acid is normally absorbed in the small intestine, you need to take a supplement formulated to allow it to reach the large bowel. As it is a dietary fat, few side-effects have been reported – but it should not be taken if you suffer from gastritis (inflammation of the stomach) or peptic ulcers.

USEFUL ADDRESSES

Please send a stamped, self-addressed envelope if writing to an organization for information.

ALLERGY SUPPORT GROUP
Little Porters
64A Marchalls Drive
St Albans
Herts
0172 758 705
Support for sufferers of any allergy.

THRUSH ADVICE BUREAU
Pre-recorded Thrush Helpline: 0171 285 5520.
For a free 16-page booklet, send a stamped, addressed A5 size envelope to: The Thrush Advice Bureau, PO Box 8762, London SW7 4ZD.

Complementary Medicine

BRITISH ACUPUNCTURE ASSOCIATION AND REGISTER
34 Alderney Street
London SW1V 4EU
0171 834 1012
Information leaflets, booklets, register of qualified practitioners.

BRITISH HERBAL MEDICINE ASSOCIATION
Sun House
Church Street
Stroud GL5 1JL
01453 751389
Information leaflets, booklets, compendium, telephone advice

BRITISH HOMEOPATHIC ASSOCIATION
27A Devonshire Street
London W1N 1RJ
0171 935 2163
Leaflets, referral to qualified homeopathic doctors.

COUNCIL FOR COMPLEMENTARY AND ALTERNATIVE MEDICINE
Suite 1
19A Cavendish Square
London W1M 9AD
0171 724 9103
Details on a variety of techniques and practices. Leaflets, booklets, newsletter.

INTERNATIONAL STRESS MANAGEMENT ASSOCIATION
The Priory Hospital
Priory Lane
London SW15 5JJ
0181 876 8261
Information on stress management and control. Leaflets, booklets, counselling.

Lapacho, Pfaffia and Guarana
For further information on these herbs from the Amazonian rainforest, contact: Rio Trading Company, 2 Centenary Estate, Brighton, East Sussex BN2 4AW; 01273 570987.

FURTHER READING

DIET AND LIFESTYLE

Leon Chaitow, *Stress* (Thorsons)
Leonard Mervyn, *Thorsons Complete Guide to Vitamins and Minerals* (Thorsons)
Stephen Terrass, *Allergies* (Thorsons)
—, *Stress* (Thorsons)

ALTERNATIVE MEDICINE

David Hoffman, *The Complete Illustrated Holistic Herbal* (Element Books)
Dr Andrew Lockie and Dr Nicola Geddes, *The Complete Guide to Homeopathy* (Dorling Kindersley)
Penelope Ody, *The Herb Society's Complete Medicinal Herbal* (Dorling Kindersley)
The Reader's Digest Family Guide to Alternative Medicine
Norman Shealy (ed.), *The Complete Family Guide to Alternative Medicine* (Element Books)
Dr Melvyn Werbach, *Healing through Nutrition* (Thorsons)
Valerie Ann Worwood, *The Fragrant Pharmacy* (Bantam Books)

INDEX

Of further interest…

RECIPES FOR HEALTH: CANDIDA ALBICANS

Featuring over 100 sugar-free and yeast-free recipes

SHIRLEY TRICKETT

Thrush, sinusitis, allergies, throat infections, depression, bloating, food cravings, weight problems, chronic muscle pain – these are just some of the conditions associated with an over-production of the yeast candida albicans in the body.

This practical self-help guide explains:

- what causes candida growth and how to prevent it
- which foods to eat and which foods to avoid

Shirley Trickett includes over 100 easy-to-prepare recipes which are low in refined carbohydrates, virtually yeast free and full of flavour, and features everyday ingredients which are readily available and economical to use.

It is a cookbook guaranteed to improve your health and well-being.

CANDIDA ALBICANS

LEON CHAITOW

Candida albicans is a yeast which exists inside all of us and normally presents no problems, but today's widespread use of broad spectrum antibiotics, contraceptive pills and steroids, as well as a sugar-rich diet, can cause a proliferation of this parasite yeast.

Its spread can often be the root cause of a wide variety of problems – ME/chronic fatigue syndrome; depression; anxiety; irritability; diarrhoea; bloatedness; heartburn; tiredness; allergies; acne; migraine; cystitis; menstrual problems, etc. Leon Chaitow shows how to detect whether yeast is your problem, and provides a comprehensive and non-drug programme for its control.

Leon Chaitow, osteopath, naturopath and acupuncturist, is a leading international practitioner and successful author of a wide range of health books.

CANDIDA ALBICANS

How your diet can help

STEPHEN TERRASS

The foods you eat and the nutritional supplements you can take may have a profound influence on your well-being. This clearly written, practical guide – based on stringent medical and scientific research – reveals how you can help yourself by explaining:

- the facts about candida albicans
- which foods to eat
- which foods to avoid
- the benefits of vitamins, minerals, herbal and other nutritional supplements

Stephen Terrass, a nutritionist and technical director for a leading vitamin company, has spent 15 years studying and researching the effects of nutritional supplementation, herbs and diet on health. He has written and narrated an award-winning series of cassette tapes which complement this Nutritional Health Series.

DIETS TO HELP: CANDIDA

The natural way to treat yeast problems

LEON CHAITOW

Thrush, chronic fatigue, allergies, anxiety, depression, bloatedness, food cravings, weight problems, chronic muscle pain – these are just some of the conditions associated with an overgrowth of the yeast candida in the body.

This book offers a full nutritional approach to managing candida albicans. Leon Chaitow clearly explains:

- what causes candida overgrowth and how to prevent it
- which foods to eat and which to avoid
- why you may need to eliminate yeast and sugary foods from your diet
- what supplements and herbs are beneficial

He includes a helpful dietary plan with delicious and easy recipes.

Leon Chaitow is a leading practitioner of osteopathy, naturopathy and acupuncture. He is the well-established author of an extensive range of health guides.

RECIPES FOR HEALTH:

CANDIDA ALBICANS	0 7225 2967 8	£5.99 ☐
CANDIDA ALBICANS	0 7225 3343 8	£3.99 ☐
DIETS TO HELP: CANDIDA ALBICANS	0 7225 3423 X	£3.99 ☐
CANDIDA ALBICANS	0 7225 3150 8	£4.99 ☐

All these books are available from your local bookseller or can be ordered direct from the publishers.

To order direct just tick the titles you want and fill in the form below:

Name: _____

Address: _____

_____

_____ Postcode: _____

Send to Thorsons Mail Order, Dept 3, HarperCollins*Publishers*, Westerhill Road, Bishopbriggs, Glasgow G64 2QT.

Please enclose a cheque or postal order or your authority to debit your Visa/Access account —

Credit card no: _____

Expiry date: _____

Signature: _____

— up to the value of the cover price plus:

UK & BFPO: Add £1.00 for the first book and 25p for each additional book ordered.

Overseas orders including Eire: Please add £2.95 service charge. Books will be sent by surface mail but quotes for airmail dispatches will be given on request.

24-HOUR TELEPHONE ORDERING SERVICE FOR ACCESS/VISA CARDHOLDERS — TEL: 0141 772 2281.